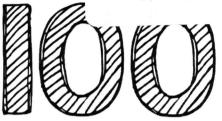

100

Acne
Tips & Solutions

The
ClearClinic
Guide to
Perfect Skin

Eric S. Schweiger, M.D., F.A.A.D.
with Melissa Schweiger Kleinman

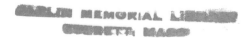

CONTENTS

Acknowledgements

Foreword by Eric Schweiger, M.D.

Acne & Acne Scar Glossary

Acknowledgements

First off we would like to thank Lauren Sundick, PA-C for her help in making this book come to life. In addition, we would like to acknowledge that parts of this book concerning skin of color and acne were written by Dr. Sejal Shah and parts concerning the emotional aspects of acne were written by clinical psychologist Dr. Laura Curtiss Feder. Thank you both for your valuable contributions. We would also like to thank our supportive team at Clear Clinic, including our wonderful physician assistants and personal acne coaches Laura Palmisano, PA-C, Diana Palmisano, PA-C, Julie Zuckerman PA-C and Jessy Ayala, PA-C. Special thanks to Wayne Westerlind and Lauren Caponong for helping with graphics, images and formatting. We would also like to thank makeup artist Maya Michelle Shapiro for lending her expertise to the book. Also, a big thank you to artist Marie Rossettie for her wonderful illustrations. We want to thank Eileen Cope for her support and enthusiasm. Also, thanks mom and dad, we couldn't have done this without you.

Foreword
by Eric Schweiger, M.D.

Jennifer came into Clear Clinic on a Tuesday. She had never had acne before and didn't know why she had been so broken out for the past three months. Her "breakout" was localized to the forehead and temples and she couldn't figure out why her skin was suddenly so bad. After photoshopping her prom pictures and faking sickness to skip out on her best friend's high school graduation party, Jennifer knew she needed help. She was well aware that her skin condition was affecting her self-esteem and her social life. With college starting just six weeks later, her self-imposed deadline for clear skin was fast approaching. Today marked her third visit to a dermatologist in three months and hopelessness was setting in.

Upon examining Jennifer at Clear Clinic, I noticed that the bumps on her face were "monomorphic." This means that all of the bumps were in the same phase of evolution, rather than appearing in different phases as acne typically presents. The truth was, Jennifer didn't have acne at all, she had a very similar-appearing condition called pityrosporum folliculitis, which occurs when yeast overgrows on the skin's surface and becomes trapped in the follicles. The tiny bumps form quickly; they resemble acne, but do not respond to acne medications or treatments.

After prescribing Jennifer a topical anti-yeast medication called ketoconazole, her bumps disappeared and she got her clear skin back in two weeks. She was able to start college looking like her old self with renewed confidence.

I wrote this book with patients like Jennifer in mind. While each patient's journey to clear skin is unique, and surely most patients' treatment takes much longer than Jennifer's, having a professional partner in your quest for clear skin is essential.

When patients come in for acne treatments, they tend to be not only concerned about their skin, but also embarrassed and ashamed of their condition. It's easy to think of acne as just a trivial, cosmetic issue. But the truth is that it has a major negative impact on those who are affected with it. While the statistics say that over 50 million people in the United States have acne at any one time, it is really 100% of people who have had to deal with it at some point in their life. Many of these people strongly feel acne goes beyond just skin deep.

This book is designed to help guide, educate and empower you when dealing with acne breakouts. Whether you have chronic cystic acne, suffer from the occasional breakout or are dealing with acne's aftermath, such as dark marks or scars, it's important to arm yourself with the right knowledge to properly address your complexion issues. I have also found that education is key when it comes to feeling better about your acne. When acne is a great unknown, it's hard to gather the right tools to fight it.

This book is broken into seven parts—in the first part, we set the record straight on the biggest acne myths and truths. Part two tells six success stories of former and current Clear Clinic patients. In the third part, we go over the biggest mistakes made by people with acne. Part four goes over the other conditions that are often mistaken for acne. In part five, we answer the 100 most common questions we've received from the thousands of acne patients we've treated over the years. Part six is a compilation of the 100 best acne-fighting tips, all of which you will find throughout the book as well. Finally, we put together a glossary of acne and acne scar terms.

My hope is for this information to be used as a resource and guide for patients with acne and should be used in conjunction with a professional partner, such as a dermatologist or other skin care specialist.

--Dr. Eric Schweiger, Clear Clinic founding dermatologist

Clear Tip #1:

Don't pop pimples at home – this can cause more inflammation on the skin.

Part 1
Acne Myths and Truths

1. Sun exposure will help clear up my complexion

MYTH: Many patients believe that their acne is improved when they have a suntan, so it is difficult for them to understand when we tell them the real answer that a suntan will not help your acne in the long term. While a tan may temporarily camouflage discoloration from old acne breakouts and can sometimes dry up excess oil on the skin, these effects are only temporary and the risk of direct sun exposure outweighs the benefits of a temporary suntan. For patients who think their skin

Clear Tip #2:

Visit your dermatologist as soon as acne develops; delaying treatment for even mild acne can lead to scarring.

gets clearer in the summer, an in-office or at home blue light therapy is a much healthier and beneficial choice.

2. Stress causes acne

TRUTH: What your mother has been telling you for so many years is actually true; stress can contribute to acne. While stress isn't the main cause of acne, increased stress can certainly make acne worse. Studies on teenagers have shown that those who were under increased stress were 23% more likely to have acne.[1] Stress causes the adrenal gland to produce excess levels of androgen and increased levels of androgen can lead to the development of acne.

3. Acne only affects teenagers.

MYTH: Although acne is most prevalent in teenagers, due to a surge of hormones that take place during puberty, many adults suffer from acne as well. On the flip side, some adult patients never had acne as a teenager.

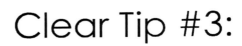

Clear Tip #3:

Laser and light treatments are great for teenagers who forget to apply medications.

4. It's OK to "squeeze" or "pop" acne lesions

MYTH: Squeezing acne lesions can lead to more inflammation and eventually scarring after the acne lesion has resolved. By popping a pimple, you can inadvertently push the bacteria further into the skin and cause even more breakouts and inflammation. At Clear Clinic, we tell our patients "bathroom surgery" is never a good idea.

5. Acne is caused by poor hygiene

MYTH: Practicing good hygiene is an important part of all skin care regimens, but many times it does not treat the underlying causes that lead to acne. Dirt itself does not cause acne.

6. Sunscreen is okay for patients with facial acne to use

TRUTH: It is actually very important for patients with acne

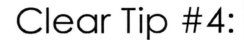

Clear Tip #4:

Wear loose, breathable fabrics while exercising or doing athletics. Tight-fitting clothing can lead to body acne.

to use sunscreens. In particular, those that are made specifically for the face and labeled "non-comedogenic" or "non-acnegenic" are best. Acne medications can make the skin more sensitive to the sun, so it's important to protect yourself from both the UVA and UVB rays.

7. I should not use moisturizer if I have acne

MYTH: Many people believe that drying out the skin is the best way to treat acne lesions, but the opposite is true. When you over-dry the skin, it tries to make up for it and produces even more oil to compensate for the lack of moisture on the skin's surface, a phenomena we call "rebound oil production." So avoiding a moisturizer can actually have the opposite effect than the one you are going for. In fact, applying an oil-free moisturizer before and after your prescription acne medications (a technique called "sandwiching") can cut down on irritation and redness.

8. Acne does not disappear overnight

Clear Tip #5:

Wash your clothes on a regular basis. Wearing the same outfit for extended periods of time may promote bacteria growth.

TRUTH: Acne takes months to develop and while medical acne treatments are very effective, they generally take around 4-6 weeks to start working. Patience is a must when it comes to treating acne. It's important to wait at least three months before deciding an acne regimen is not working for you.

9. Laser acne treatments work quickly

TRUTH: Laser acne treatments work more quickly for the treatment of acne than prescription treatments. Laser and light treatments such as photodynamic therapy and Isolaz® can help to improve acne within a few weeks.

10. Acne scars can improve when treated

TRUTH: Laser treatments for acne scarring, such as the fractional CO2 laser and the fractional Erbium Glass laser (Fraxel® laser), are very effective for the treatment of acne scarring. Our F.A.S.T.® (Focal Acne Scar Technique) procedure treats patients with localized acne scars with the fractional CO2 laser then the Fraxel®

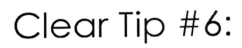

Clear Tip #6:

Washing with a salicylic acid cleanser after working out can help to prevent body acne.

laser with great results and reduced recovery time.

11. Acne is treated differently in every patient

TRUTH: It is important to see a skin care professional to determine the right course of treatment for your particular type of acne. Some examples of treatments include topical creams, prescription face washes, oral antibiotics, oral anti-androgen treatments or birth control pills in women, laser treatments and light treatments.

12. Acne can be caused by hormones

TRUTH: Hormones called androgens can cause increased sebum production in the sebaceous glands. This is why stress, certain foods, pregnancy and menstrual cycles, all of which can trigger an influx of hormones in the body, can contribute to acne breakouts.

13. It is a good idea to put toothpaste on a pimple overnight

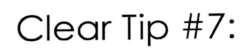

Clear Tip #7:

Make sure to change your pillowcase every day when acne is a consideration. Dead skin cells, dirt and debris accumulate on the pillowcases and can lead to more breakouts.

MYTH: This popular home remedy is not recommended. Not only can toothpaste cause irritation to the skin, it can actually contribute to the formation of new acne. The best spot treatment for acne is a cortisone injection into the pimple, which can flatten it within 24 hours.

14. You Cell Phone Can Cause Acne

TRUTH: The more you talk on your phone with it pressed up against your face, the more likely you will breakout in that area. Holding your phone against your skin can cause oil to get trapped in the pores, causing pimples. Try using earphones instead or wash your face after a long conversation.

15. Use more acne products for faster results

MYTH: In this case, less is more. Using too much of your topical acne medications can cause excessive irritation on your skin, in the form of redness and peeling. A pea-size amount is sufficient for treatment of your entire face; you should use much less if applying only to spots. Don't forget to moisturize after medication application!

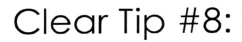

Clear Tip #8:

If you're running out of clean pillowcases, then use a clean t-shirt as a pillowcase alternative.

16. It's ok to apply makeup to cover up acne

TRUTH: It is safe to apply concealer or foundation to cover up acne on your face. You should choose makeup labeled as non-comedogenic, which means that it will not contribute to the formation of acne. At the end of the day, be sure to remove your makeup before you go to sleep.

17. There is no need to treat teenage acne, as teenagers "grow out of their acne"

MYTH: It is important for all people, including teenagers, to treat acne promptly when it develops. If left untreated, acne can become more severe and cause pitted scars. The medications and treatments used to treat acne are safe for teenagers; there is no need to wait for teenagers to "grow out of their acne."

18. You should stop acne medications once your skin is clear

MYTH: Nearly all acne sufferers should continue at least

Clear Tip #9:

Use a white pillowcase if you use benzoyl peroxide at night; it can bleach fabric, but won't bleach your skin.

some of their acne medications once their acne has cleared. Acne is a chronic condition, meaning that it can last a very long time and takes a long time to develop. It is not something that just "goes away" with treatment. Often the influencing factors behind the acne are still present, and the acne clearance can be maintained with the simple application of a once-daily cream.

19. Your diet can play a role in acne

TRUTH: While the common thinking among many skin care specialists has been that diet does not play a large role in the presence of acne, recent research and studies in this area are rocking the boat on this perception. A report from the American Academy of Dermatology found a low-carbohydrate, low-glycemic diet, such as the South Beach Diet may in fact help reduce acne. Low glycemic foods include fresh fruit and leafy green vegetables as well as whole grains, lean meats, whole milk and minimally processed foods. In the study, 80% of South Beach Diet followers noticed a marked improvement in their skin within three months of beginning the diet, while 91% of them said they were

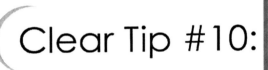

Clear Tip #10:

Avoid hairstyles that require a lot of hair product, as oils can clog pores.

even able to decrease the acne medication they were taking after starting the diet[2]. The thinking behind these findings is that a high-glycemic diet triggers a hormonal response in the body that results in the production of more sebum, which leads to acne.

20. You should avoid Accutane® at all costs

MYTH: Accutane® is the closest thing that we have to a cure for acne and it is the right medication for those patients who need it.

Clear Tip #11:

If you're using hairspray or other product on your hair, sleep with a headband on to keep it off your face.

PART 2
Clear Clinic Patient Stories

At Clear Clinic, it's our job to listen to patients. There is no "one-size-fits-all" treatment plan for acne and to get the best results we partner with our patients to find a plan of action that works best for both their skin and their schedules. Oftentimes a patient will come to us after several failed attempts at fixing their skin on their own or with another doctor. Our approach includes a comprehensive strategy that best fits the needs and goals of each patient. Hearing about others' success is

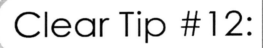

Clear Tip #12:

A low glycemic diet may help to reduce acne. Cut back on processed foods and add more leafy green vegetables and berries to your diet.

sometimes the best motivator of all. In that respect, we'd like to share some of our patients' stories with you. From a thirty something wanting to get rid of her acne scars before her wedding to a recent college graduate looking for acne treatments that are covered by insurance, here are their inspiring stories.

1. 31-Year-Old Female with Hormonal Acne

Patient: Diana, a 31-year old healthy female who came in for treatment of acne breakouts on her chin.

Her story: For Diana, the sudden appearance of acne on her chin was very frustrating and embarrassing. Throughout her teenage years, Diana's skin was always clear. She wasn't used to wearing makeup to cover up her acne and desperately wanted to get her old skin back. Six months prior to her appointment with us, she had taken Doxycycline 150mg and used a benzoyl peroxide/clindamycin combination gel for three months without significant improvement of her acne. She rarely had acne on her cheeks or forehead, the acne flared only on her chin. More specifically, Diana experienced a cystic acne flare on her chin each month a few days prior to her period and the cysts would persist

Clear Tip #13:

Choose organic milk when possible, there is less of a chance that the cow has been injected with hormones, which could potentially lead to acne breakouts.

throughout the rest of the month. Three months prior to her Clear Clinic appointment, Diana began taking the oral contraceptive pill Ortho Tri-Cyclen. She estimated that she experienced 50% improvement after starting the pill, though her premenstrual flares still continued.

Clear Clinic treatment: After an evaluation at Clear Clinic, Diana began taking a low dose of an anti-androgen medication called Spironolactone, which blocks excessive androgen influence in female patients. Spironolactone does have some potential side effects including increased urination and occasional irregular periods or breast tenderness. Diana experienced no side effects while on the medication. After six weeks, Diana saw a significant improvement in her premenstrual breakouts. After three months, Diana was no longer experiencing any routine premenstrual breakouts and was completely clear and she tapered off to topical maintenance.

2. 25 Year Old Male With a 12-Year History of Acne

Patient: Alan, a 25-year-old healthy Hispanic male with

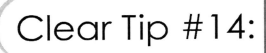

Clear Tip #14:

Adults with acne can benefit from a retinoid—it helps treat acne and wrinkles.

a history of acne on his face for twelve years.

His story: Prior to visiting Clear Clinic, Alan had used numerous topical acne medications including clindamycin gel, tretinoin, tazarotene, and salicylic acid. Alan was frustrated with the process and sick of trying new topical medications every few months with little improvement. He was also concerned about the red marks left behind after the acne bumps ran their course.

Clear Clinic treatment: On his first visit to Clear Clinic, Alan began a series of laser and light treatments, which included Isolaz® treatments, photodynamic therapy treatments, and red and blue light treatments. He also restarted using a clindamycin/benzoyl peroxide 1%/2.5% combination gel each night. His first in-office procedure was with the Isolaz®, a treatment that combines a vacuum for pore cleansing with a broad-spectrum light to kill the P. acnes bacteria. When Alan returned to Clear Clinic one week after his Isolaz® treatment, he had already experienced an improvement in his active acne, though he was still developing new acne. On his second visit, photodynamic therapy (PDT) was performed. Photodynamic therapy uses a

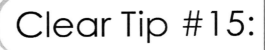

Clear Tip #15:

Wear sunscreen daily while taking oral antibiotics for acne.

The Clear Clinic Guide to Perfect Skin

medication called aminolevulinic acid, which is activated by blue light, to kill the P. acnes bacteria and decrease sebum production. Alan experienced mild redness and peeling for three days after the photodynamic therapy though was able to continue his normal work and social obligations. He was careful to avoid sun exposure for 48 hours after the treatment, as PDT makes your skin very sun sensitive for that time.

On his third visit, Alan had red and blue light therapy, which provides anti-inflammatory and anti-bacterial influence without the downtime of a PDT treatment. Light therapy can help to decrease post-inflammatory erythema (the redness left behind after acne) in addition to treating and preventing acne. Alan had a second PDT on his fourth visit and a second Isolaz® treatment during his fifth visit, five weeks after initially coming to Clear Clinic. During this time, Alan continued to apply benzoyl peroxide/clindamycin gel each night. After his fifth week of treatment, Alan no longer had any active acne on his face.

Two years after Alan completed our physical acne treatment program, his face has remained clear

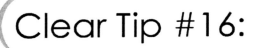

Clear Tip #16:

For sun protection, we recommend using a physical sunblock containing zinc oxide or titanium dioxide; chemical sunscreens are more likely to irritate.

of acne. He continues to use the benzoyl peroxide/ clindamycin 2.5%/1% cream each night, and comes in every six months for one maintenance photodynamic therapy session.

3. 27 Year Old Female with Acne Scars

Patient: Marisa is a 27-year-old female who came to our office with deep-pitted acne scars on her cheeks.

Her Story: Marisa had severe acne in high school, but had not had any active acne for over 15 years. Marisa was very bothered by her acne scars; her wedding was approaching in six months and she was concerned that makeup would not distract from the appearance of the pitted scars on her cheeks. Two years prior, Marisa had received Restylane® injections into the pitted scars, she liked the appearance immediately after the Restylane® injections, but felt that the improvement wore off too quickly. She now wanted a permanent solution for her acne scars.

Clear Clinic treatment: After a discussion of treatment options, Marisa decided to have F.A.S.T.® fractional

Clear Tip #17:

If you have a pimple and need it gone fast, see your dermatologist for a cortisone injection, which can flatten your pimple in 24 hours, and is usually covered by insurance.

CO2 laser resurfacing. The Focal Acne Scar Treatment (F.A.S.T.®) technique treats a focused area of acne scarring rather than the whole face. Marisa felt that F.A.S.T.® fit her schedule best, as she only needed to take a few days off of work to recover.

The F.A.S.T.® procedure was performed on a Wednesday afternoon; Marisa took Thursday and Friday off from work for recovery. Marisa arrived in the office one hour prior to her treatment for numbing. A topical anesthetic cream was applied to her face for one hour. The laser treatment itself took approximately 20 minutes and Marisa felt no pain during the treatment. Immediately after the treatment, she applied ice for a few minutes and reviewed post-treatment care with Dr. Schweiger. Aquaphor® ointment was applied to the treated skin and Marisa went straight home.

After four days of relaxing at home, Marisa had only mild redness on her skin, which was easily covered with light makeup. She returned to Clear Clinic one week after her treatment. Her skin was healing well and both Dr. Schweiger and Marisa estimated a 30-40% improvement of her acne scars after just one week. Full

Clear Tip #18:

Stress can be a contributor to acne outbreaks. Try to exercise on a daily basis. A workout, when combined with meditation or some other form of relaxation, can help decrease stress.

collagen regeneration takes up to six months. After three months, Marisa was seeing nearly 60% improvement in the depth of her acne scars. On her wedding day, Marisa's makeup went on smoothly and she felt very happy about her laser resurfacing results.

4. 22 Year Old Female with Severe Acne

Patient: Jamie, a 22-year-old female who has been battling severe acne for years.

Her story: Prior to coming to Clear Clinic, Jamie took oral antibiotics and used what felt to her like "every topical medication out there" for acne. No treatment had ever helped her in the past. She was incredibly frustrated and felt that she would have acne forever. She came to us two months after graduating college. As a new graduate looking for a job, she wanted to stick with treatments that were covered by insurance so lasers weren't an option. In addition, she felt that she needed to clear up her skin in order to feel more confident as she interviewed for jobs.

Clear Clinic treatment: During her first visit, Jamie

Clear Tip #19:

If it doesn't seem like acne, it might actually be something else such as rosacea or Pityrosporum follicultitis. Talk to your dermatologist about other diagnoses that look similar to acne.

inquired about taking Accutane®. After a long consultation, Jamie decided to enroll in iPledge, which is the governing body of Accutane®. iPledge requires that every female patient taking Accutane® have two negative pregnancy tests, 30 days apart, prior to starting Accutane®. Jamie took a urine pregnancy test in the office; the test came back negative and she was enrolled in iPledge. Jamie came back to the office 30 days after her initial appointment. She had a second negative pregnancy test at this visit and was now ready to begin Accutane®. In her first month of taking the medication, Jamie had no adverse effects besides mild dry lips, though she saw no improvement of her acne. Like many patients, Jamie did not see improvement of her acne until her third month of Accutane® treatment. It was around this same time that she began to notice very dry skin and extremely chapped lips. This improved somewhat after beginning a good moisturizing regimen for both her skin and lips. Other than excessive dryness, Jamie had no side effects from Accutane®. She did not experience mood changes, GI distress, or muscle aches, although these are a few of the potential side effects to watch out for while taking Accutane®.

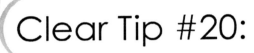

Clear Tip #20:

Blue and red light therapy are safe and effective acne treatment options during pregnancy.

After six months of Accutane® treatment, Jamie had reached the required total dose of medication for her weight. Jamie no longer was having acne flares and had not had any new acne for over two months. She stopped taking Accutane® and began using a topical retinoid for maintenance. One month after stopping Accutane®, Jamie had her last pregnancy test and no longer needed to check in with iPledge. She was also completely clear for the first time in over seven years.

Jamie had a very positive Accutane® experience, as most patients do. She felt confident and was able to find a job while taking the medication. Her only regret was that she did not take Accutane® years before, when her acne was at its worst.

5. 14 Year Old Female with Comedonal Acne

Patient: Samantha is a 14-year-old female who presented with mild acne on her forehead.

Her story: She developed acne only a few months prior to her visit, but was very embarrassed by it and wanted to get rid of it as quickly as possible. Samantha's mom

Clear Tip #21:

Glycolic and lactic acid cleansers can safely be used during pregnancy.

came with her to the visit. They had tried Proactiv® and over-the-counter salicylic acid cleansers, but none of the over-the-counter treatments helped significantly. Samantha's mom tried to convince her to grow out her bangs, because she felt her hair was contributing to her forehead acne, but Samantha refused. She used the bangs as a device for covering her acne.

Clear Clinic treatment: Dr. Schweiger examined her skin and realized that most of Samantha's acne was comedonal, meaning that she predominantly had blackheads and whiteheads (as opposed to pink papules, or bumps). Samantha was a busy teenager, so her mom worried that numerous acne medications to use at home might be burdensome and difficult to use. After discussing potential treatment options, it was decided that Samantha would begin a series of medical extractions to quickly clear up the comedones on her forehead. She would follow a simple regimen at home, using the Clarisonic brush for two minutes each morning in the shower with an over-the-counter salicylic acid acne cleanser to thoroughly clean out her pores and tretinoin gel in the evening to reduce comedone formation on her forehead.

Clear Tip #22:

Acne-like bumps on the beard are not always acne – it may be a condition called pseudofolliculitis barbae. Consult your dermatologist if you're not sure.

Samantha had her first medical extraction treatment prior to leaving the office that day. Our licensed esthetician steamed her pores for a few minutes prior to extracting her blackheads and whiteheads, which took approximately 30 minutes. When she left the office, Samantha had significantly fewer comedones on her forehead than when she walked in. She began using the Clarisonic brush and tretinoin gel at home that evening, which helped to clear up the remaining comedones.

Samantha continued her simple at-home regimen of the Clarisonic brush and tretinoin gel. The regimen was easy to use and didn't take much time out of her day. Once every three to four months, Samantha comes into Clear Clinic for a medical facial, to keep her pores clear. She continues to also use tretinoin gel nightly at home and continues to do well.

6. 40 Year Old Female with Mild Acne

Patient: Kelly is a 40-year-old female who came in with mild acne on her face.

Her story: Kelly was frustrated and embarrassed and

Clear Tip #23:

Less is more: even over-the-counter formulations can cause excessive dryness if overused. Take a few days off from your acne products if you develop redness or irritation.

felt that as a 40-year-old, she should be more concerned with anti-aging and wrinkle prevention than treating acne. She wanted to clear up her acne in order to start using anti-aging creams and improving fine lines and sun spots that had developed on her skin over the years.

Clear Clinic treatment: It was explained to Kelly that many people have acne in their adult years. The fortunate thing is that some of the medications that we use for acne treatment can have anti-aging properties as well. The class of medications known as retinoids helps fight the signs of aging as well as prevent acne breakouts. Retinoids, which are the only anti-aging product that has also been FDA approved to reduce the formation of fine lines and wrinkles, are also an effective acne medication. It was explained to Kelly that retinoids stimulate skin cell turnover, which decreases the microcomedone formation in the follicle that attracts the P. acnes bacteria that causes acne. In addition, it stimulates collagen production, which softens fine lines and prevents the formation of fine lines in the future.

Kelly began using a retinoid called tazarotene. Initially, she experienced mild redness and peeling,

Clear Tip #24:

Look at your skin care products and if they contain fragrance it may be time to look for a different brand. Synthetic fragrances contain many ingredients that may be irritating to your skin.

but when she began to use a smaller amount of the medication and combine it with a light moisturizer before and after the medication, this irritation subsided. One month after starting tazarotene, Kelly was not only noticing improvement of her mild acne, but she felt that her skin was smoother and looked healthier. Even some of the dark sun spots were starting to lighten.

For the first time in years, Kelly felt that her acne was under control and she could finally focus on anti-aging.

Clear Tip #25:

Make sure all of your skincare products say "non-comedogenic" or "non-acnegenic" on the label somewhere.

Part 3
The Top 10 Mistakes People With Acne Make

Mistake 1: Picking or popping your acne

This leads to increased inflammation, which in turn means a greater risk of scarring. The increased inflammation can also mean a pimple that sticks around way longer than invited. Instead of picking, visit your dermatologist for a quick cortisone injection, which flattens acne in 24-48 hours.

Clear Tip #26:

Use a pea-size amount of your acne medication, to minimize risk of skin irritation and apply to the whole face: cheeks, forehead and temple. Don't just spot treat!

Mistake 2: Stopping your regimen too soon

Acne can take months to respond to any medication or skincare regimen. Do not assume that if you're not clear after 2 weeks that the medicine is not working. Continue all treatments for at least 8 weeks before you decide it's not working.

Mistake 3: Using too many acne treatments

Using too many products at once can be a problem. We recommend that our patients using prescription medications for acne use very gentle cleansers and moisturizers. If cleansers and moisturizers with active ingredients are used in combination with prescription treatments, the result can be increased irritation.

Mistake 4: Using too much of an acne medication, or using it too often

This may cause irritation to the skin. It is better to use

Clear Tip #27:

Apply moisturizer before and after using a topical retinoid. This technique is called "sandwiching" and helps cut down on irritation to the skin.

only as much of the medication as you can tolerate, and eventually increase the frequency of use. Many patients use too much and then stop the treatment before it has a chance to work. Same goes for spot treatments – if you use too much of a spot treatment, it can in turn cause irritation and inflammation, which can lead to pigmentation or redness after the acne resolves.

Mistake 5: Washing too aggressively

There is no need to over-wash your acne prone skin. Washing too often or too aggressively can cause irritation and excessive dryness. Washing twice daily with a gentle cleanser is sufficient.

Mistake 6: Avoiding moisturizers

Many patients with acne feel that using a moisturizer will make their skin too oily and cause more acne. This is false; if you use a moisturizer that is made for acne prone skin (labeled "non-comedogenic" or "non-acnegenic"), it can actually protect the skin and can prevent irritation

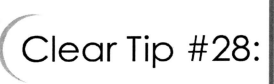

Clear Tip #28:

Apply retinoids in the evening to reduce sun sensitivity.

from acne treatments. In addition, if your skin is too dry, it may actually cause the sebaceous glands to increase oil production, which makes your skin more greasy.

Mistake 7: Tanning

"Will going to the tanning bed help?" is a question that we are frequently asked in the office. The answer is an emphatic "no." While some light treatments benefit acne, we never recommend tanning. The main reason not to go tanning is that recent studies have linked UV exposure in tanning beds to an increased risk of melanoma, that deadliest form of skin cancer.

Mistake 8: Waiting to see a dermatologist

We often see patients with severe acne scarring, who have never seen a dermatologist. Had they seen a dermatologist earlier in the course of their acne, much of the scarring could have been avoided. Dermatologists treat even very mild acne and know how to make a regimen specifically for your type of acne breakout.

Clear Tip #29:

While taking Accutane, apply Aquaphor® ointment liberally to your lips, to avoid excessive dryness.

Mistake 9: Stopping acne treatments as soon as the skin is clear

Nearly all acne sufferers should continue at least some of their acne medications once their acne has cleared. Acne is a chronic condition, meaning that it can last a very long time and takes a long time to develop. It is not something that just "goes away" with treatment. Often the influencing factors behind the acne are still present, and the acne clearance can be maintained with the simple application of a once-daily cream.

Mistake 10: Avoiding Accutane® at all costs

Accutane® is a necessary and actually a wonderful medication for the right patient. Many patients walk into the office and say "there is no way I will ever use Accutane®." While we feel that Accutane® is not a first line therapy, it is a viable option for severe acne that is not responding to other treatments. We recommend our patients stay open to this possibility. Accutane® is the closest thing that we have for an acne "cure" and it is a great medication for those patients who need it.

Clear Tip #30:

Use an at-home blue light device between in-office blue light treatments for best results.

Part 4
Rosacea and Other Acne Imitators

Sometimes what appears to be acne is not actually acne. There are conditions that resemble acne, but are not acne so must be treated differently to be successful. Many such patients that visit the Clear Clinic have tried acne medications for these conditions in the past, without any improvement. Once a proper diagnosis is made and treatment initiated, most patients will see a great improvement in the appearance of their skin.

Clear Tip #31:

Avoid sun exposure for 48 hours after photodynamic therapy.

Rosacea: Rosacea is an inflammatory condition that is commonly mistaken for acne. It can sometimes look very similar to acne, with reddish bumps on the cheek, though it can also present with simply redness and telangiectasia ("broken blood vessels") on the skin. Notably, rosacea does not have blackheads or whiteheads. There is no known cause for rosacea, though it is theorized that demodex mites, which live in the hair follicles, may play some role in its development. Certain environmental triggers, such as heat, spicy foods, and alcohol, can cause rosacea to flare.

Rosacea can be treated with prescription medications and in-office laser treatments. Prescription medications used for the treatment and management of rosacea include topical metronidazole and azeleic acid, sodium sulfacetamide/sulfar formulations, and low doses of doxycycline. A new topical medication called Mirvaso®, immediataley cuts down the redness associated with rosacea. "Erythrotelangiectatic rosacea" (rosacea that is composed mostly as redness and blood vessels) generally requires treatment with a vascular laser, such as the KTP laser or the VBeam laser. These lasers help to collapse the superficial blood vessels that contribute

Clear Tip #32:

Use a foaming cleanser that doesn't need to be rubbed into the skin to lather. Rubbing the skin can cause further irritation.

to the appearance of redness. Patients may see signs of improvement after a short series of treatments.

Pityrosporum Folliculitis: Pityrosporum folliculitis is another condition commonly mistaken for acne. Pityrosporum folliculitis presents as tiny papules (skin-colored or reddish bumps) and pustules (pus bumps) on the face, chest and back. They are "monomorphic," meaning that all of the bumps look the same. In the case of acne, the bumps are at many different stages at any given time. This is one of the giveaway features of pityrosporum folliculitis.

Pityrosporum folliculitis is caused by a type of yeast that is regularly found on the skin's surface. Some people react to this yeast by forming these small bumps on their skin. Anti-yeast medications are used in the treatment of pityrosporum folliculitis, in order to decrease the colonization of yeast on the affected area.

Follicular Eczema: Follicular eczema is a skin condition resulting in the appearance of itchy, rough bumps around the hair follicles. These bumps can sometimes

Clear Tip #33:

Don't do bathroom surgery! Rather than perform extractions at home, book an appointment with a medically trained skincare professional who uses sterile tools to minimize risk and maximize results.

resemble acne to an untrained eye. We recommend that our patients who are prone to follicular eczema moisturize regularly with a hydrating cream. Prescription medications are usually required for treatment of a follicular eczema flare; we often prescribe topical steroid creams to be used for a short period of time.

Sebaceous Gland Hyperplasia: Sebaceous gland hyperplasia is commonly seen on the forehead and nose, in a similar distribution to acne. These bumps are caused by overgrowth of the sebaceous (oil-producing) glands on the skin. Sebaceous gland hyperplasia appears as soft, yellowish bumps that do not resolve on their own. Sebaceous gland hyperplasia is not dangerous, though some of our patients find it to be unsightly. In-office procedures, such as Photodynamic Therapy (PDT), electrocautery, and laser resurfacing, can be used to reduce the appearance of sebaceous gland hyperplasia.

Pseudofolliculitis Barbae: Many of our male patients experience pseudofolliculitis barbae (referred to as PFB)

Clear Tip #34:

Stay away from spa facials where the esthetician is massaging oils and heavy creams into your face.

on their beard area. They tell us that acne bumps form on their neck when they shave. PFB forms when coarse, curly beard hairs reenter the skin and cause irritation to the follicle this results in the formation of inflammation around the hair follicle. PFB can sometimes be managed with a specific shaving regimen, though often prescription medications are necessary.

Acne Keloidalis Nuchae: Acne keloidalis nuchae (AKN) is a condition seen in African American men. The most common area for AKN to present is the back of the scalp and neck. The bumps of AKN begin as skin-colored or reddish bumps at the nape of the neck, but quickly progress to form keloid-type scars. Although AKN has "acne" in its name, it is actually not a form of acne at all. In order to properly treat AKN, both the initial bumps and the keloid scars must be treated. Common treatments for AKN include antibiotics, topical steroids, retinoids, and intralesional steroid injections to flatten the raised keloid scars.

Keratosis Pilaris: Keratosis pilaris is a condition

Clear Tip #35:

If you have a tendency to pick and squeeze your pimples, avoid looking into mirrors during the day.

commonly seen on the upper arms, though it can also form on the thighs, buttocks, and face. Many people believe that they have formed acne on their arms, but this is often not the case. Keratosis pilaris presents with very tiny, reddish bumps that form as a result of keratin plugs in the hair follicles. Keratosis pilaris is not dangerous, but many of our patients wish to improve its appearance. The most common treatments for keratosis pilaris include topical urea and glycolic acid, both of which reduce the excess keratin plugging the hair follicle. Lasers can also be used to treat keratosis pilaris; vascular lasers can provide an improvement of the reddish appearance.

Clear Tip #36:

Wash your washcloths often so you're not touching your skin with bacteria trapped in the towel.

PART 5
100 Acne
Questions & Answers

1. What causes acne?

For acne lesions to form several factors have to come into play, "the perfect storm" so to say. The first step of acne development is the formation of the microcomedone, which is a microscopic form of a pimple and cannot be detected by the naked eye. The microcomedone forms as a result of abnormal regulation of the cells within a hair follicle. Most people don't realize it, but everyone's body is covered by tiny little microscopic

Clear Tip #37:

Make sure to wash your hands before applying your makeup. The oils and bacteria on your fingers may be contributing to your acne breakouts.

hair follicles. There are over 5,000,000 hair follicles on the human body and only about 100,000 of those follicles are on the scalp. The only areas that do not have hair follicles are the palms, soles, lips and genitals. Many of these hair follicles are tiny and don't produce a visible hair. When a microcomedone forms on a hair follicle (often one on the face that does not produce a hair), dead skin cells and sebum are unable to leave this pore. This collection is an ideal environment for the propionbacterium acne (P. acnes) bacteria to flourish. You may not be aware of it, but the P. acnes bacteria lives on the surface of everyone's skin and only becomes an issue when the pores become clogged and it gets trapped. This clogging causes the P. acnes bacteria to get caught inside the pore, where it eats the sebum then flourishes, creating inflammation and eventually leading to an inflammatory acne lesion (aka a zit).

Clear Tip #38:

Don't sleep in your makeup. If you're too tired to wash your face, use a makeup remover pad.

The progression of a pimple

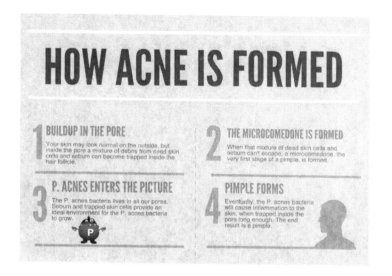

HOW ACNE IS FORMED

1 BUILDUP IN THE PORE
Your skin may look normal on the outside, but inside the pore a mixture of debris from dead skin cells and sebum can become trapped inside the hair follicle.

2 THE MICROCOMEDONE IS FORMED
When that mixture of dead skin cells and sebum can't escape, a microcomedone, the very first stage of a pimple, is formed.

3 P. ACNES ENTERS THE PICTURE
The P. acnes bacteria lives in all our pores. Sebum and trapped skin cells provide an ideal environment for the P. acnes bacteria to grow.

4 PIMPLE FORMS
Eventually, the P. acnes bacteria will cause inflammation to the skin, when trapped inside the pore long enough. The end result is a pimple.

2. Do hormones play a part of the development of acne?

Yes, sex related hormones called androgens can contribute to the development of acne. In particular, androgens can increase the production of sebum (skin oil). Each hair follicle on your body has an associated sebaceous gland (oil gland). These oil glands were put on our body to help us. They make sebum, which naturally protects and hydrates the skin. These oil-

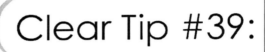

Clear Tip #39:

Wipe your cell phone down daily with an alcohol swab to kill any bacteria and reduce oils that may get transferred onto your skin.

producing glands are also sensitive and responsive to androgens and when the body has an excess of androgens it's like giving the oil glands a green light to produce more sebum. It's when the skin sebum levels go up that you run into problems. Sebum is like a candy for the P. acnes bacteria; they eat it and grow off it. As sebum production increases, so does the proliferation of P. acnes bacteria and in turn acne breakouts. This is why one of the ways we treat acne is trying to decrease skin sebum levels.

3. Does acne run in families (is it genetic)?

A gene causing acne has not yet been found, but evidence shows us that acne likely has some genetic predilection. We find patients with a family history of severe acne are more likely to have severe acne themselves. But just because your mom or dad had acne, does not mean that you have to just accept fate. There are many actions to take to treat and manage acne breakouts regardless of family history. With the right knowledge, treatments and products, you do not need to let history repeat itself.

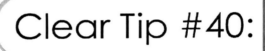

Clear Tip #40:

Swap your cream blush for a powder blush. Cream formulations are more likely to consist of pore-clogging ingredients.

4. At what age do people usually first develop acne?

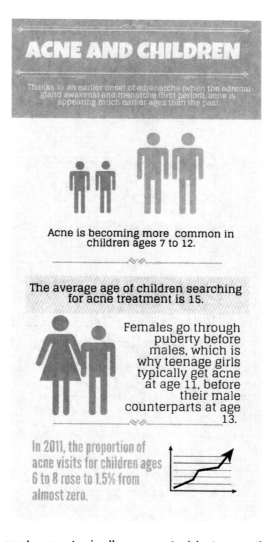

ACNE AND CHILDREN

Thanks to an earlier onset of adrenarche (when the adrenal gland awakens) and menarche (first period), acne is appearing much earlier ages than the past.

Acne is becoming more common in children ages 7 to 12.

The average age of children searching for acne treatment is 15.

Females go through puberty before males, which is why teenage girls typically get acne at age 11, before their male counterparts at age 13.

In 2011, the proportion of acne visits for children ages 6 to 8 rose to 1.5% from almost zero.

In the past acne typically presented between the ages of 11 and 13, correlating with puberty, but according to a new set of guidelines regarding acne treatment in

Clear Tip #41:

Make sure to wash your makeup brushes on a regular basis to clear them of bacteria and debris that can lead to acne breakouts.

children published in the May 2013 issue of the journal Pediatrics, acne is common in children ages 7 to 12. Thanks to the earlier onset of adrenarche (when the adrenal gland awakens) and menarche (first period), acne is appearing at much earlier ages than years past. A 2011 study in Pediatric Dermatology, which assessed an estimated 93 million physician visits for acne by children 6 to 18, the average age for seeking acne treatment has decreased slightly, from 15.8 in 1979 to 15.0 in 2007[1]. The proportion of acne visits by children 6 to 8 rose to 1.5 percent from practically zero. Teenage acne often presents earlier in females than males, with males first getting acne closer to 13 years of age and females around 11 years of age. This is because females usually go through puberty before males.

5. How common is acne?

It's nice to know that you're not alone in your fight against acne. There are many people with acne; in fact, over 50 million people in the United States have acne. Nearly 85% of people between 12-24 years of age develop acne to some degree. It is said that 100% of people will experience an acne breakout of at least a few pimples at

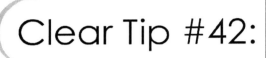

Clear Tip #42:

Stop using retinoids three days prior to laser scar resurfacing treatments.

some point in their life.

6. Are there different types of acne?

Yes, the main two categories of acne are "inflammatory" and "non-inflammatory" acne. Non-inflammatory acne lesions are blackheads and whiteheads, officially open and closed comedones, respectively. Inflammatory acne is what is traditionally thought of as pimples and cysts. Inflammatory acne lesions can lead to scarring.

7. Is acne contagious?

No, acne is not contagious. The P. acnes bacterium is not infectious in the same way as other bacteria. Acne is your body's reaction to the P. acnes bacteria, in addition to other factors, such as increased sebum production. You cannot catch acne from someone else.

8. What sunscreens are best for patients with acne prone skin?

The variety of sunscreens available at your local drugstore can often be intimidating. There are many great sunscreens for people with acne-prone skin, but it is important to know what you are looking for.

Clear Tip #43:

Visualize a stop sign to help yourself put the brakes on negative thoughts about yourself.

Patients with acne are often using acne medications, such as retinoids or oral antibiotics, which make their skin more susceptible to sunburn. In-office procedures for the treatment of acne, such as photodynamic therapy, also make the skin very sensitive to the sun. The most important thing for a patient with acne to look for when purchasing a sunscreen is the phrase "non-comedogenic" or "non-acnegenic." This means that the sunscreen has been tested and proven not to contribute to the formation of acne lesions. Mineral sunblocks may also be less irritating to acne-prone skin than chemical sunscreens. It is important that the sunscreen provide both UVA and UVB protection.

9. Do teenagers outgrow their acne?

As teenagers grow older, their hormones and the hormonal influences on their skin change. Usually acne decreases as the androgenic influence of puberty decreases in the late teens and early twenties. However, hormones are not the only cause of acne, and some teenagers do not see improvement in their acne as they get older. In addition, some people get acne for the first time in their twenties, after never having acne in high

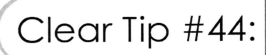

Clear Tip #44:

Don't use your fingertips to wash your face, as bacteria lurking under the nail can aggravate acne.

school. It is important to treat acne promptly whenever it presents; simply waiting to outgrow acne can lead to permanent scars and years of active acne.

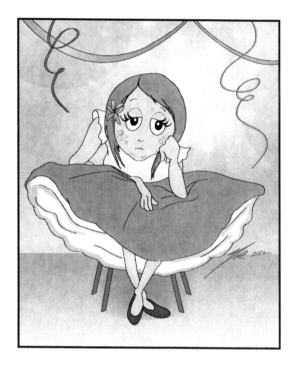

10. I'm a parent, how can I talk to my teen about seeking treatment for acne?

It's most likely that your teen feels self-conscious about their skin if they're suffering from acne. Start by asking your child how his or her skincare has been going and if they are looking for any help with it. A recent study showed that most teens do not seek medical help for

Clear Tip #45:

To avoid skin picking, time yourself in the bathroom so you're not allowing yourself extra time to pick.

their acne. The best way to get your teen the help they need is by making them an appointment with a dermatologist. Stress to them how important it is to take good care of their skin and that a dermatologist is just like any other doctor they would see. The skin can get sick, too and a dermatologist will help find the right treatment to make it better.

11. How common is adult acne?

According to reports, adult acne is on the rise, especially in females. Studies have shown that up to 50 percent of women between the ages of 20-29 have acne as well as up to 25 percent of women ages of 30-49 are affected with acne.[2], [3] Hormones are big culprits for these breakouts. When women get older, their levels of androgens can surge. This hormone surge can play a large role in sebum production and how quickly the skin sheds its cells, which can lead to acne flae-ups. Rosacea is another skin issue that needs to be addressed, as many people often mistake it for acne.

Clear Tip #46:

Avoid touching your face when working or studying for exams. Face touching leads to breakouts.

12. Is there a difference between adult acne and teenage acne?

The same causative agents that lead to acne formation form both adult and teenage acne. At Clear Clinic we notice adults have drier skin, so we often avoid prescribing medications that are overly drying in our adult population. We also prescribe our adult patients an acne-fighting medication with anti-aging benefits, such as retinoids. For these reasons, it is best to use a gentle but still effective treatment regimen for adult acne patients.

13. What else may be causing my adult acne breakouts?

Adults with acne who have it localized to their forehead and trunk, especially when all of the bumps look the same may have not have acne at all. Rosacea and pityrosporum folliculitis may be other diagnoses to consider. Pityrosporum folliculitis is an acne imitator caused by yeast on the skin. These patients respond better to oral and topical anti-fungal medicines than they do to anti-acne medications. Patients we have seen at Clear Clinic like this are amazed when their acne-like

Clear Tip #47:

Wash your hands before washing your face.

bumps go away after only a few weeks of treatment. Often they have tried at home acne medications for some time without success before seeing a dermatologist. Sometimes even dermatologists don't think of this diagnosis, so feel free to bring it up at your appointment.

14. What is rosacea?

About 16 million Americans have rosacea, yet very few seek the proper treatment for it. In fact, many people mistake rosacea for acne. Like acne, rosacea is an inflammatory condition. Rosacea may present itself in many ways, the most common being acne-like bumps on the face and erythema (redness) with telangiectasia (blood vessels.) The exact cause of rosacea is unknown and there is no cure. Rosacea may be worsened by certain triggers, which can differ in every patient. Vasodilation, which is a flushing on the face, is exaggerated in patients with rosacea upon exposure to heat.

15. What is the difference between acne and rosacea?

Acne and rosacea are different conditions, with different causes, though they appear very similar. Rosacea

Clear Tip #48:

Strongly consider Photodynamic Therapy or Accutane® if you have severe acne.

bumps can mimic acne, often making it very difficult to distinguish the two conditions from each other. However, patients with rosacea do not develop comedones (blackheads and whiteheads), and acne patients do not experience flushing. These are two key ways to differentiate the two. Also, rosacea is more common on the central face—cheeks, nose and chin.

16. What is acne keloidalis nuchae?

Acne keloidalis nuchae, a condition commonly seen on our African American patients, is when firm bumps appear at the posterior hairline. Many people mistake this for acne vulgaris (aka acne). Keloidalis refers to its scar-like nature and "nuchae" means neck. The truth is acne keloidalis nuchae is actually not acne at all. It is really a bunch of circular keloid scars that have formed around the hair follicles in this region. We do not know why it occurs, presumably due to a folliculitis-like condition (inflammation of the hair follicles) on the scalp. Folliculitis can occur from friction, follicle blockage or shaving.

17. How do you treat acne keloidalis nuchae?

Acne keloidalis nuchae is treated by a variety of

Clear Tip #49:

Remember that even celebrities get acne. Cameron Diaz, Annalynne McCord, Kate Hudson have all had bouts with acne.

methods. The bumps of acne keloidalis nuchae can be treated effectively with intralesional steroid injections. This helps to flatten out the bumps on the scalp. Topical and oral antibiotics, as well as topical steroids can be used to treat AKN and prevent new bumps in the future. The good news is that patients usually respond quite well to aggressive treatment.

18. How common is it to feel depressed if you suffer from acne?

It is very common for acne sufferers to feel depressed. In a variety of studies, anywhere from 13-38% of acne patients—or as high as half of adolescent acne patients—report depression or meet criteria for other psychological disorders[4],[5]. Low self-esteem, anxiety, social stigmatization or isolation and feelings of helplessness and hopelessness—all symptoms of depression—can be side effects that accompany acne. There is an increased correlation between depression and acne, but correlation does not indicate causation. A complicating factor is that the time that is most common for acne to strike, late adolescence and early adulthood, is also a very common time for psychological

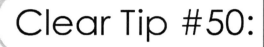

Clear Tip #50:

Don't fight acne alone—partner with a skincare professional, such as a dermatologist.

symptoms to emerge. If you are experiencing feelings of depression, consult with your doctor immediately.

19. What can I do to prevent myself from picking at my acne?

If a simple admonition from yourself, a person close to you or a doctor does not get you to stop picking at your acne by simply telling you, you may be suffering from a skin-picking condition called neurotic excoriation. These are called body-focused repetitive-behaviors (BFRBs): repetitive self-grooming behaviors in which pulling, picking, biting or scraping of the hair, skin or nails result in damage to the body. These troubles can be similar in certain ways to obsessive-compulsive disorder and often include elements of perfectionism. Those with BFRBs often experience a physical or emotional urge to pull or pick and a feeling of tension or boredom commonly triggers the behavior, resulting in fleeting pleasure, gratification or relief while engaging in the pulling/picking that quickly can turn to self-directed anger or guilt afterward. With BFRBs often comes shame, secrecy, isolation, and interference with intimate relationships, avoidance of activities one would otherwise pursue as

Clear Tip #51:

Don't waste your time on microdermabrasion if you have deep pitted scars.

well as possible interference with work or study.

If self-help is not enough and you believe you are suffering from a skin-picking disorder or other BFRB, we suggest counseling. The website www.trich.org is a great resource to learn more and to help find a qualified mental health professional to help you stop picking.

20. How is acne different in patients with skin of color?

Acne in skin of color is very similar to acne in patients with lighter skin types. Acne breakouts occur from the same factors, regardless of your skin tone. However, treating acne can present some unique challenges for patients with skin of color. Patients with skin of color are prone to residual dark marks for weeks to months after acne breakouts. These left over marks are called "post-inflammatory hyperpigmentation" (PIH), which can be very difficult to treat and frustrating for the patient.

21. Can using hair oils cause acne?

Hair oils have become increasingly popular in the United States in recent years. They can potentially cause

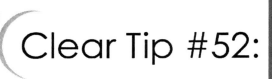

Clear Tip #52:

If your skin is feeling dry, skip your acne medications for a day then restart. (Don't forget to moisturize though).

acne around the hairline because they are usually comedogenic, meaning that they can clog up the pores and lead to the formation of the microcomedone, which causes acne. Using hair oils on the scalp does not cause acne everywhere, but it can contribute to acne formation on adjacent areas where the hair touches, such as the forehead and upper back.

22. How common is new onset acne when you are pregnant?

Acne is a very common skin complaint we see in our pregnant patients. Whether you had acne prior to becoming pregnant or begin breaking out once you conceive, it's very typical for women to experience breakouts due to the hormone fluctuations taking place. We observe that the most common time for expecting women to breakout is during the first trimester.

23. If you get new onset acne when you are pregnant how soon does it resolve after you give birth?

The period after giving birth is often referred to as the

Clear Tip #53:

Rosacea patients can often benefit from sulfur-based washes.

"fourth trimester" because of all the changes still taking place in your body. After giving birth, the hormone levels in your body can be unpredictable for a few months, so you can still expect acne flares during this time. Our patients often notice reduced acne starting after three to four months post-delivery. But this can vary greatly.

24. What are the best acne treatments for teenagers that don't require a prescription?

While there is no one "best' non-prescription acne treatment, there are several available effective topical treatments for teenagers. These treatments include salicylic acid, benzoyl peroxide, sulfur, green tea and tea tree oil. The ideal regimen may include a combination of these ingredients and is different for each individual patient.

25. How does salicylic acid work?

Salicylic acid is a "keratolytic agent," meaning it's a peeling agent that helps remove the top layer of the skin. Salicylic acid also helps shed cells inside the hair follicles, which in turn prevent the pores from clogging and keeps them free of debris. Salicylic acid can help

Clear Tip #54:

Always give your new acne regimen at least 2 months to work before you change it.

reduce whiteheads and blackheads. Salicylic acid concentrations approved for use in over the counter treatments for acne fall between 0.5 percent to 2 percent. The negative side of salicylic acid is that it can cause stinging and skin irritations, such as cracking and redness.

26. How does benzoyl peroxide work?

After all of these years, benzoyl peroxide still remains one of the top acne medications. Available in both over-the-counter and prescription formulations, it is a treatment that nearly everyone with acne has tried at some point. Benzoyl peroxide works by adding oxygen to the pores, which kills the bacteria responsible for acne (Propionibacterium Acnes). Like salicylic acid, benzoyl peroxide also helps clear the pores of cellular debris. Benzoyl peroxide products generally come in non-prescription concentrations of 2.5 percent, 5 percent and 10 percent. Side effects can include dryness, redness and flaking. There is evidence that 2.5% benzoyl peroxide actually has the same effectiveness as 10%, just with decreased side effects.

Clear Tip #55:

Keep a diary of past medications so you will be able to look up what worked and what didn't in case you forget (as everyone does).

27. Can your skin get used to acne medications? Is it important to continually change your regimen?

It is unlikely that your skin "gets used to" or becomes immune to acne medications, though the needs of your skin may change over time. The acne regimen that worked great last year may need to be tweaked as your skin changes this year. Acne often responds well to changing medications every so often, though it is unlikely that this is because the acne has become "used to" the medication.

28. What should I do if others start making fun of my acne?

Feeling good, strong and centered about oneself regardless of outside comments or influences is the antidote in this situation and the key to "thicker skin." In addition to tuning out such negative noise as teasing or nasty comments, it may help to think about what may be going on with those who are making fun of you.

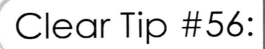

Clear Tip #56:

Use mineral based make-up to cover up an outbreak.

29. Should people with acne-prone skin use a moisturizer?

The answer is yes, absolutely. Many patients with acne prone skin skip moisturizing because they feel that the more they "dry out" their skin, the fewer acne lesions they will have. The truth is that some acne patients do have excessive oil production from their sebaceous glands; however, this does not necessarily result in moisturized skin. Under-moisturizing can also result in "rebound" oil production, which makes your skin even oilier. In addition, many acne medications, including over-the-counter spot treatments can be irritating and drying, so it is important to keep acne-prone skin hydrated. Once patients with acne prone skin realize that they need to be moisturizing regularly, they often have questions about the best moisturizer for their skin type. It is important that patients with acne-prone skin look for moisturizers with the phrases "non-comedogenic," "non-acnegenic," or "oil-free" on the label. These phrases indicate that the moisturizer should not to contribute to the formation of acne.

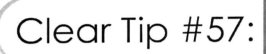

Clear Tip #57:

Men can use tinted moisturizer to cover up a break out.

30. Do at-home blue light devices work as well as in-office treatments?

While in-office blue light treatments are stronger than at-home blue light devices, the at-home devices certainly serve a purpose in a good acne-fighting regimen. They can be well utilized in between office visits as maintenance therapy. We find that patients with busy schedules who cannot make it into the office for regular in-office treatments often turn to at-home blue light devices. Blue light acne therapy targets the root cause of acne, the P. acnes bacteria that lives in the pores. As the non-UV blue light waves shine on the acne bacteria cells, it actually kills them! The most effective treatment regimen is often a combination of in-office blue light treatments and at-home blue light treatments.

31. In what order should I apply my topical treatments?

This is a very common question we get from patients and it can get very confusing, trying to figure out the order of application. While the order can vary depending on what's in your regimen, typically it should look something like this:

Clear Tip #58:

Don't stop using acne medications just because you are clear.

Step one: Cleanser

Step two: Light oil-free moisturizer

Step three: Topical treatment medications and spot treatments

Step four: Light moisturizer (often with sunscreen for morning regimen)

Step five: Makeup (optional)

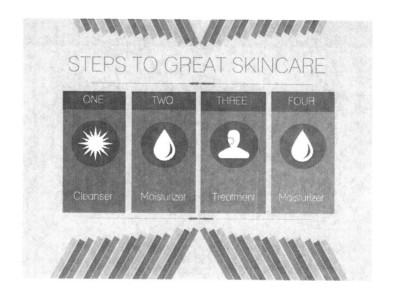

Clear Tip #59:

Hormonal acne in females can often be treated successfully with birth control or Spironolactone (both are prescription, so see your doctor!)

32. How are antibiotics used to treat acne?

Antibiotics are commonly used in the treatment of inflammatory acne, which is when your body's defense system produces an inflammatory response to the P. acnes bacteria trapped in the pores, thanks to a traffic jam of oil, hair and dead skin cells. Inflammatory acne presents as red, inflamed pimples with no white or blackhead. Antibiotics can be used topically in the treatment of mild to moderate inflammatory acne or taken by mouth for the treatment of moderate to severe inflammatory acne. Antibiotics work in a few different ways to reduce acne. The main mechanism that antibiotics use to treat inflammatory acne is to decrease the amount of P. acnes bacteria around the pore. Antibiotics also work by reducing the concentration of free fatty acids in the sebum; free fatty acids promote inflammation and may cause comedones (whiteheads and blackheads).

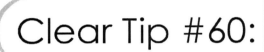

Clear Tip #60:

Laser Genesis is a good treatment for mild acne scars.

33. What are some examples of topical antibiotics used to treat acne?

The most common topical antibiotic used in dermatology today for the treatment of acne is clindamycin. Clindamycin directly targets the P. acnes bacteria that cause acne. Clindamycin is frequently combined with benzoyl peroxide in what is called a "combination medicine." This combination works better than either product alone. Common prescription combo medications include Duac®, Benzaclin® and Acanya®. These combination formulations have been clinically shown to be superior to either individual ingredient on their own. In recent years, clindamycin has also been combined with tretinoin. Other topical prescription antibiotics used to treat acne include, the antibiotic Erythromycin and Dapsone.

34. Are topical antibiotics just as good as oral antibiotics?

Depending on the severity of your acne, your dermatologist may decide to give you a topical antibiotic, an oral antibiotic or both. Topical antibiotics are sufficient for the treatment of acne in many patients. However,

Clear Tip #61:

Not all fractional lasers used for treating acne scars are the same. Make sure to ask your dermatologist the difference before you get treatment.

patients with more severe acne may need an oral antibiotic. Topical antibiotics treat and kill the bacteria on the skin from the outside in, while oral antibiotics kill the P. acnes bacteria from inside the pores. Topical and oral antibiotics are often used in combination with other medications in order to get optimal results.

35. What are the most effective oral antibiotics for the treatment of acne?

As with topical medications, there is no one oral medication that is necessarily "best." The medication most often prescribed will vary based on the type of acne and the patient's lifestyle. The "tetracyclines" are the most commonly prescribed oral antibiotics for the treatment of inflammatory acne. These include the medications doxycycline and minocycline. The tetracyclines work by interfering with bacterial protein synthesis and kill the P. acnes bacteria. Examples of doxycycline and minocycline are the brand names Doryx® and Solodyn®. Most studies have shown all antibiotics to be of relatively equal effectiveness, although some may work better on particular people for unknown reasons.

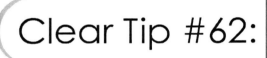

Clear Tip #62:

Do not wait to "outgrow" acne, seek treatment now.

36. What are the side effects of oral antibiotics?

All oral antibiotics have unique side effects; your dermatologist can review the potential side effects for the oral antibiotic that you are taking. Side effects that are potentially seen with most antibiotics used for acne are stomachaches, headaches, dizziness and vaginal yeast infection.

37. How long does it take to see results from prescription medications?

Topical prescription medications take approximately one month to begin working. Oral prescription medications tend to work more quickly, usually within two weeks for patients to start to see improvement.

38. If the oral antibiotic works, do I have to stay on it forever?

No, the current recommendations for treatment suggest limiting oral antibiotic use to three to six months and then transitioning to topical medications for "maintenance therapy"[6]. We find that this strategy works very well for the treatment of acne and prevents side effects from long-term antibiotic use.

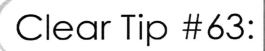

Clear Tip #63:

One size does not fit all for acne treatment. Make sure you have a customized regimen.

39. Do oral antibiotics make me more sensitive to the sun?

Yes, many oral antibiotics are light-sensitizing, meaning that you are more likely to get sunburned if you are taking them. Doxycycline is the most light-sensitizing of all the oral medications commonly used for acne treatment. This means it is very important to use sun protection or avoid the sun when on this medication.

40. Will being on an oral antibiotic make me resistant to this antibiotic if I need it in the future?

This is a common question we get from patients and the answer is no it will not. Individual patients do not become immune to the affects of one antibiotic just because they are on it for a long period of time.

41. What is Retin-A?

Retin-A is a brand name of tretinoin, one example of a topical retinoid. This class of medication regulates skin cell turnover and helps to prevent formation of the microcomedone in the skin follicle. Formation of a microcomedone attracts P. acnes bacteria, so by

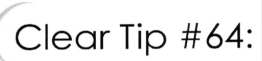

Clear Tip #64:

Keeping pictures of your face can be a great way to track your progress.

preventing the microcomedone, retinoids decrease the formation of acne lesions.

42. Are acne treatments anti-aging?

One of the benefits of using a topical retinoid medication to treat acne is that it also helps the skin retain a youthful look. Topical retinoids regulate skin cell turnover while helping remove the acne-causing microcomedone from the follicle. Simultaneously, the same medication works to stimulate collagen production in your skin, which leads to smoother skin and fewer fine lines in the future. Retinoids are an important part of many acne regimens. Patients receive the anti-aging benefit of the medications at the same time as the anti-acne benefit. When combined with a great sunscreen and moisturizer, retinoids provide a fantastic anti-aging regimen with no extra effort.

43. How do I reduce dryness caused by my topical retinoid medications?

Tretinoin and other retinoids are great treatments for both acne and anti-aging. However, we often hear the complaint that these treatments can be irritating. If used

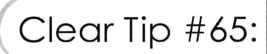

Clear Tip #65:

Check out ClearTrack™ at www.clearclinic.com to easily track your progress on your way to clear skin.

improperly, they can cause excessive redness and even peeling. We recommend using retinoids only three nights a week initially, and starting Monday-Wednesday-Friday. With time, the frequency of use can be increased without having increased irritation. To minimize irritation, we recommend applying moisturizer immediately before and after the retinoid, so-called "sandwiching", and using only a pea-sized amount of the medication. If irritation occurs after applying a retinoid, (this is called "retinoid dermatitis"), there are a few things that can be done to improve the appearance of the skin quickly: Stop using the medication for a few days, as the skin is healing. You may apply over-the-counter hydrocortisone twice daily for up to five days and use as a gentle moisturizer. Once the skin has healed, you may restart the retinoid slowly.

44. What is Accutane®?

Isotretinoin is the generic name of the drug better known as Accutane® (we will refer to it as Accutane in this book). Accutane® treats acne by a number of mechanisms, including decreasing sebum production by permanently modifying the sebaceous glands, regulation of skin cell

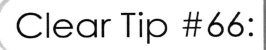

Clear Tip #66:

Avoid alcohol if you are taking oral antibiotics or Accutane®.

turnover and reduction of skin inflammation.

45. Is Accutane® safe?

When properly monitored and prescribed by an experienced medical professional, Accutane® can be a safe and effective medication. While it is true that Accutane® has many potential side effects, many of these can be limited by monthly monitoring of labs. There are some serious potential side effects that patients need to be aware of before starting Accutane®, but most of these side effects are very rare. Often the effectiveness of the treatment will outweigh the potential side effects.

46. Is Accutane® safe for teenagers?

Teenagers with severe acne that has not responded to other treatments may be appropriate candidates for Accutane® therapy. Accutane® has many potential side effects but when properly managed can be a safe and effective medication. Some teenagers should not begin taking Accutane® until they are fully grown. In some instances, Accutane® has been shown to prematurely stimulate epiphyseal (growth plate) closure and decrease cartilage formation. Your dermatologist and pediatrician

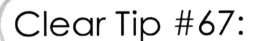

Clear Tip #67:

If you are overweight, try to get back to your ideal weight. Obesity is associated with increased acne.

will work together to determine when and if Accutane® is an appropriate treatment for your acne. Many teenagers do very well after taking Accutane® and avoid permanent scarring from uncontrolled acne. Patients who are not appropriate candidates for Accutane® therapy, but whose acne has not responded to other medications, often do very well with laser and light-based treatments for acne.

47. What is the most common side effect of Accutane®?

The most common side effect of Accutane® is excessive dryness of the skin and lips, which is found in the majority of patients.[7] Patients may find that their lips and skin are very dry; we recommend using moisturizers and emollients on the lips (Vaseline works very well) and body regularly to address this issue. Other, more rare side effects include gastrointestinal and liver damage.

48. Does Accutane® lead to depression?

There have been reports that link Accutane® (isotretinoin) with mood changes, depression and even

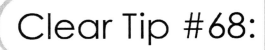

Clear Tip #68:

Seeking aggressive treatment for acne early can decrease the chance of having scars later.

suicide in patients. While these symptoms must always be taken seriously by patients, families and doctors, it is a complicated clinical picture. Depression and its associated symptoms are related to acne in terms of a vicious cycle often involving low self-esteem, feelings of helplessness and hopelessness, a lack of control, anxiety and stigmatization or self-imposed isolation. Complicating this is the likelihood of acne to strike during adolescence, a time of great emotional flux and insecurity as well as a high prevalence of psychological symptoms. It should be noted that no studies have been able to demonstrate Accutane® causing an increase in depression or suicidal behavior. In fact, some recent studies have shown exactly the opposite. A 2010 review of over 1700 patients taking Accutane® showed no increased incidence of suicidal ideation or attempted suicide.[8] A 2011 study suggested that, in fact, it is severe acne that should be linked to increased depression, and not Accutane® usage.[9] This sentiment was also reflected in a 2012 study, which showed that psychological disturbances were clearly increased by acne, but not by Accutane®.[10] For patients with a history of depression, we often recommend meeting with a mental health

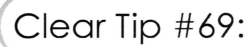

Clear Tip #69:

Consider a Fraxel® treatment if you have post-inflammatory hyper-pigmentation (residual dark spots after acne resolves).

professional prior to starting Accutane®. However, recent clinical studies illustrate the safety of Accutane® for most patients.

49. Why does Accutane® have such a bad reputation?

Accutane® certainly receives a lot of bad press. This negative perception is likely due to its long list of potential (and rare) side effects. Because of its potential side effects, Accutane® is used as a "last resort" medication. It is used for severe resistant acne that has not responded to other treatments. However, an overwhelming majority of acne patients have a positive experience with acne and experience lifelong reduction in acne breakouts after taking the medication.

50. Does Accutane® always work?

Most patients do very well after taking a full course of Accutane®, with about 95% responding positively. Accutane® is a weight-based medication, meaning that a course of Accutane® is completed once the patient has taken a certain amount of medication per pound of weight. Patients who complete the appropriate

Clear Tip #70:

Both green tea and tea tree oil are good natural ingredients that may help fight acne.

dose usually are happy with the results. Unfortunately, there are still a very small percentage (about 5%) of patients who do not experience clearance of acne after taking Accutane®. For most patients, Accutane® is a "cure," meaning that they never have acne again. After completing Accutane®, people still get occasional pimples, but they don't usually get severe breakouts like they did prior to taking Accutane®. For some patients, they are clear for many years after taking Accutane®, but they do flare at some point in the future. The good news is that after taking Accutane®, most patients respond better to conventional acne medications and do not need to restart Accutane®. Some patients do not experience clearance of their acne while taking Accutane®, but this is the minority of patients. Most patients do very well after Accutane® treatment. Patients who respond well to Accutane®, but have an acne flare a few years later may benefit from a second course of Accutane®. This is safe and often effective.

51. How long does Accutane® take to work?

Accutane® is usually taken for a course of approximately

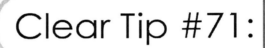

Clear Tip #71:

Consider KTP laser treatment if you have red marks from old acne.

six months. It is a pill that is usually taken once or twice daily with food. Some patients notice improvement immediately, while other patients actually notice that their acne gets worse briefly before getting better. Most patients see an improvement in their acne by the second or third month of treatment.

52. I thought that Accutane® went off the market, is this true?

No, this is false. The brand name "Accutane®" medication is no longer manufactured. This was a business decision and not a result of being "pulled from the market" or anything similarly dramatic. Isotretinoin (the generic form of Accutane®) is still available in several generic formulations. The names of these generic medications include Sotret®, Amnesteem®, Claravis®, and Myorisan®.

53. Can I take Accutane® during the summer?

Accutane® may be taken during the summer months, though patients must be diligent with sun protection. Accutane® makes your skin more sun sensitive, so regular sun protection and avoidance of excess direct sunlight is recommended.

Clear Tip #72:

If you decide to do laser resurfacing for acne scars, give yourself about 7 days to be out of sight if you can.

54. Can I drink alcohol while taking Accutane®?

Alcohol should be avoided while taking Accutane®. A possible side effect of Accutane® is liver complications. Since alcohol is known to damage the liver, the combination of alcohol and Accutane® could be twice as harmful to the liver.

55. How long do I have to wait until I can have children after taking Accutane®?

Female patients must wait one month after finishing Accutane® before trying to conceive. Each month, female patients will have a pregnancy test prior to starting their next Accutane® prescription. There is a final pregnancy test that is administered one month following the last dose of Accutane®.

56. Does Accutane® cause permanent gastrointestinal problems?

A very rare potential side effect of Accutane® is an increased risk of developing inflammatory bowel disease. This risk is increased with higher doses of Accutane® treatment, though current Accutane® treatment

Clear Tip #73:

Your acne does not need to be completely clear before treating scars.

recommendations use lower doses than in previous years. In a 2010 study, increased doses of Accutane® resulted in increased risk of ulcerative colitis. There was no increased risk of Crohn's disease.[11] Although the risk of gastrointestinal effects is quite low, it is important to discuss any history of gastrointestinal disease with your dermatologist prior to starting Accutane®, in order to determine whether Accutane® treatment is a safe option for you.

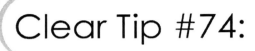

Clear Tip #74:

Chemical peels are not usually the best treatment for deep acne scars.

The Scoop on Accutane

What is accutane and is it safe?

What is accutane?

Accutane is the brand name of a generic medication called isotretinoin, which treats acne by decreasing sebum production, regulating cell turnover and reducing skin inflammation.

What are the side effects of Accutane?

Most patients experience dry lips and dry skin. Rarely more serious side effects can occur such as liver damage and bowel problems. It is important to be under the care of a licensed medical professional when taking Accutane.

Who should take Accutane?

Patients with moderate to severe acne that have not responded to other treatments are good candidates for Accutane. Although younger patients who are not fully grown and women looking to become pregnant should not take Accutane.

How long does Accutane take to work?

Accutane is typically taken for six months. While some patients notice improvement right away, others may experience more breakouts before the effects begin to take shape. Most all patients see an improvement in their acne by the second or third month of treatment.

Clear Tip #75:

If you use benzoyl peroxide, make sure it is micronized. It can then be absorbed better.

57. What are some strategies to boost my self-esteem when I have a bad breakout?

The first step is to notice and track your thoughts, particularly such negative ones such as "my acne makes me ugly." Then develop strategies and other "self-talk statements" where you can talk back to and "reframe" negative thoughts to more positive, self-nurturing statements. For example: " My acne is so low on the list of what makes me who I am. I am an awesome friend and a great dancer." Optimally, this results in feeling better, which affects your behavior – thoughts, feelings and behavior are all related and improvements to one often lead to improvements in the other. To follow this example, going out with friends and dancing provides ways to distract oneself from negative thoughts about acne, reminds one of all of the great and fun other stuff in life and reinforces positive thoughts and feelings about oneself.

58. What should I look for in makeup formulations if I have acne-prone skin?

The general rule for choosing makeup for acne prone skin is the fewer the ingredients, the better. Look for

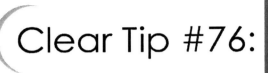

Clear Tip #76:

If you have dry skin, use a moisturizer cream; if you have oily skin use a moisturizer lotion instead.

makeup that is labeled fragrance-free, hypoallergenic, non-acnegenic, non-comedogenic, and are powder-based. Mineral makeup usually contains less chemicals and extraneous ingredients than most cosmetics, and does not need as many preservatives as liquid cosmetics, since it comes in powder form. Once you add water into a product, you need preservatives in it to prevent bacteria from forming.

59. Is there any truth to the myth that chocolate causes acne?

There have been a few studies looking at chocolate and acne. It has long been considered a myth that chocolate causes acne, and most dermatologists would agree that it does not. At least two studies have found no correlation between eating chocolate and experiencing acne breakouts. But there was a small study released in 2011 that actually found an increase in breakouts after pure chocolate consumption.[12] While this study was small (only 10 patients) and consisted only of men, it may add some controversy to the acne and chocolate debate. We personally feel that chocolate does not

Clear Tip #77:

Consider a live video chat with a Personal Acne Coach™ if you do not have easy access to a dermatologist: www.clearclinic.com.

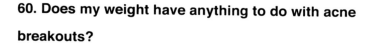

contribute to acne formation.

60. Does my weight have anything to do with acne breakouts?

While an unhealthy diet may not be a major reason for acne breakouts, it turns out weight may play a role in clear skin. In a recent study in The Archives of Dermatology, researchers looked at 3,600 adolescents and found that the overweight or obese teens had more potential to develop acne than did teens of normal weight. This was especially true for the young women. Researchers say that androgens might be to blame for the link between being overweight and acne, as androgen production is brought on by obesity[13].

61. Is it true that sugar and dairy will make breakouts worse?

Traditional medicine tells us that sugar and dairy do not affect acne. However, recent studies have shown that sugar and dairy may influence the development of acne. Interestingly, in countries that consume a low glycemic and low-dairy diet, acne is less common. Of course, there are other factors that may come into play, but this

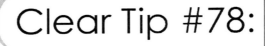

Clear Tip #78:

Don't share acne medications with your friends.

leads researchers to believe that sugar and milk do play a role. Other studies have shown that consumption of dairy may result in hormone signaling that leads to the development of acne.

62. Does a high-glucose diet play a part in acne breakouts?

More evidence that diet may play a role in acne management is from a report from the American Academy of Dermatology that found a low-carbohydrate, low-glycemic diet, such as the South Beach Diet, might in fact help reduce acne. In the study, 80% of South Beach Diet followers noticed a marked improvement in their skin within three months of beginning the diet, and 91% of them said they were able to decrease the use of their acne medications after starting the diet.[14]

Clear Tip #79:

F.A.S.T.® Laser Treatments are a great way to reduce acne scars. Patients can fly into NYC for treatment and have their travel costs included: www.flyinforclearskin.com.

63. What are some examples of high-glycemic foods?

Foods that are considered high on the glycemic index (GI) are the processed, simple carbohydrates such as white bread products, cookies, candy, white rice, white potatoes and breakfast cereals. When a food registers high on the GI, it means that its carbohydrates break down quickly and release glucose into the bloodstream at a faster pace than other foods.

THE ACNE FOOD PYRAMID

A low glycemic diet may help to reduce acne. Cut back on processed foods and add more leafy green vegetables and berries to your diet.

Eat and drink organic whenever possible.

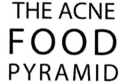

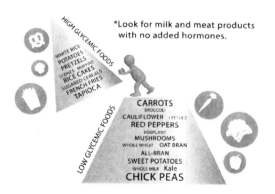

HIGH GLYCEMIC FOODS

*Look for milk and meat products with no added hormones.

WHITE RICE
POTATOES
PRETZELS
SCONES MUFFINS
RICE CAKES
SUGARED CEREALS
FRENCH FRIES
TAPIOCA

LOW GLYCEMIC FOODS

CARROTS
BROCCOLI
CAULIFLOWER   LETTUCE
RED PEPPERS
EGGPLANT
MUSHROOMS
WHOLE WHEAT   OAT BRAN
ALL-BRAN
SWEET POTATOES
WHOLE MILK   Kale
CHICK PEAS

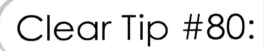

Clear Tip #80:

If you are on Benzamycin,® keep it in the fridge or it will stop working as well after a few weeks.

64. Does drinking milk affect my acne?

There has been new research linking milk—especially skim milk—to acne breakouts. A recent article in the Journal of the American Academy of Dermatology stated that there is an association between milk consumption and acne. The claim comes from a study performed at the Harvard School of Public Health of 47,000 women. The study states: "We found a positive association with acne for intake of total milk and skim milk. We hypothesize that the association with milk may be because of the presence of hormones and bioactive molecules in milk."[15] It's long been known that hormones are injected into the cows to make them produce more milk. And since hormonal activity is one of the reasons we breakout, it's an easy parallel to draw. Also, much of the milk we drink comes from cows who produced it while pregnant, which leads to the presence of even more hormones.

Clear Tip #81:

Do not use expired acne medication, if it is old throw it out!

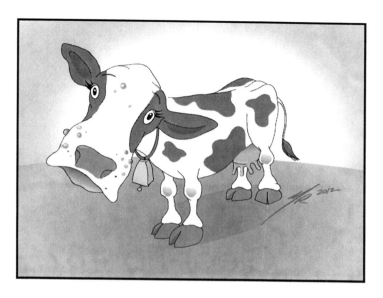

65. Can oral contraceptive pills help to treat adult acne?

Oral contraceptive pills can be effective in treating adult acne in female patients. A few oral contraceptive pills, such as Yaz and Yasmin, have an FDA indication for the treatment of acne, though many oral contraceptive pills may be beneficial when treating female adult acne. However, women who are hoping to become pregnant soon should look for an alternative treatment for fighting acne.

The best and most effective ways to treat acne in women in their childbearing years are often through blue

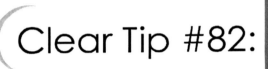

Clear Tip #82:

If you pick your skin and it starts bleeding put aquaphor ointment on the wound to prevent a scab from forming. (And try not to do that again!)

light therapy, cortisone injections, Isolaz® laser treatments and Category B prescription topical medications, such as azeleic acid. Category B medications are generally considered safe in pregnancy and nursing.

66. Does LED light help to treat adult acne?
Red and Blue LED light can be used to treat adult acne, both at home and in the doctor's office. Red and Blue LED lights are anti-inflammatory and anti-bacterial. There is no downtime after the treatment. These treatments are often combined with other therapies and prescription medications.

67. What is a cortisone injection and should I be getting them?
Cortisone injections are an in-office procedure administered by a dermatologist and a terrific option for those who want an acne lesion to disappear quickly. Cortisone injections contain a low concentration of an anti-inflammatory medication called Triamcinolone, which is a steroid medication, (a type of cortisone.) It is injected right into the acne lesion while it is flaring. Over the next 24-48 hours, the anti-inflammatory effects of

)(Clear Tip #83:

Make sure you have a spot treatment in your regimen.

Triamcinolone take effect and the acne lesion will flatten out. Most inflammatory acne lesions can be treated with a cortisone injection.

68. What are medical extractions?

During a session of medical extractions, a licensed esthetician may steam your skin for a few minutes to open up your pores. The esthetician will then clean out your clogged pores, eliminating your comedones (whiteheads and blackheads). Medical extractions are appropriate for most acne patients; they are often performed in conjunction with other in-office acne treatments and acne medications. Medical extractions are often combined with chemical peels, in order to achieve the most improvement. You may notice some redness of the treated area after your extractions, but you may apply makeup if desired. Most patients go back to work or social activities immediately following the treatment.

69. Do you recommend seeing an esthetician for medical extractions on a regular basis?

Yes, especially if you are prone to picking at or popping

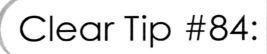 Clear Tip #84:

We often recommend patients with chronic psuedofolliculitis barbae (razor bumps) to consider laser hair removal as a permanent treatment option.

your own acne. So another question you might be thinking is what makes a medical extraction different than using your own two fingers to pop a zit (something we at Clear Clinic refer to as "bathroom surgery" and is a big no-no)? The answer is a lot. First, popping your own zits is never a good idea. It can lead to further breakouts, scars and irreparable damage. Plus, the chances of you being able to fully remove the blemish without a medical tool is very low.

70. Does intense pulsed light (IPL) help active acne?

Yes, intense pulsed light (IPL) has been shown to help both active acne and the scarring that remains after acne lesions clear[16]. Also known as photofacials, IPL uses a broad spectrum of light to target melanin (the pigmented cells forming sun spots and pigmentation after acne lesions) and hemoglobin (the red cells that are found in blood vessels and redness that remains after acne lesions.) Red and brown marks on the skin can be greatly reduced after a series of IPL treatments. A series of three or four treatments is generally required for the best results. The treatments should be spaced three to five weeks apart.

Clear Tip #85:

A monthly mask can sometimes boost your acne-fighting regimen!

71. What is photodynamic therapy?

Photodynamic therapy (PDT) is a non-invasive treatment that utilizes a blue light to activate a medication called 5-aminolevulinic acid. PDT works to reduce acne by two separate mechanisms. First, it shrinks the sebaceous (oil-producing) glands of the skin. This reduces acne by decreasing the amount of oil in each pore (remember, the P. acnes bacteria loves to eat oil!). Photodynamic therapy also directly targets the P. acnes bacteria that lives on the skin surface and causes acne breakouts. After PDT treatments, the overall texture of the skin is usually improved. In addition, we find that PDT helps post-inflammatory erythema and post-inflammatory hyperpigmentation (the red and brown marks that linger after acne lesions).

72. What is Isolaz®?

The Isolaz® treatment is an in-office procedure that is used to clear out your pores and kill the P. acnes bacteria that leads to acne. There are two components to the Isolaz® treatment, a gentle suction that cleans your pores, and a light that simultaneously destroys

Clear Tip #86:

Do not pick at your skin if it is flaky from too much medication use. Instead use extra moisturizer that day.

the P. acnes bacteria. A 2008 study showed that acne continued to improve for three months following a series of Isolaz® treatments[17]. The same study showed a decrease in both inflammatory (pimples) and non-inflammatory (blackheads and whiteheads) acne and reported that 82% of patients were moderately to very satisfied with their treatment.

73. Are laser and light treatments safe during pregnancy?

There are no studies linking laser or light treatments to birth defects, and logically speaking laser light is similar to light from a light bulb in a lot of ways, so it should not harm the fetus. We often treat patients with blue and red light during pregnancy as long as their OB/GYN is also on board and approves the treatment.

74. What is the SmoothBeam® laser?

SmoothBeam® is a laser treatment that uses thermal energy to decrease oil production from sebaceous glands. The non-invasive laser is performed in a series of treatments. The resulting decreased sebaceous gland activity causes the P. acnes bacteria to be less attracted

Clear Tip #87:

Acne can occur on the buttock and legs, and those areas often do well with a benzoyl peroxide wash.

to the follicles, which decreases the development of acne.

75. What is a chemical peel?

A chemical peel is a procedure performed in a doctor's offices with the goal of improving acne, acne scars, and/or marks from old acne spots. During a chemical peel treatment, a peeling agent, such as glycolic acid or salicylic acid, is applied to the skin for a brief period of time to remove the top layer of skin. A chemical peel helps remove dead skin cells, which can help prevent clogging of the pores. There are several chemical peels used for acne treatment, including Jessner's Peel, glycolic acid peels and salicylic acid peels. Our favorite chemical peels for acne are the Jessner's Peel and 30% salicylic acid peels.

76. What is microdermabrasion?

Microdermabrasion is an in-office treatment that removes the outer layer of dead skin cells. The procedure uses a gentle mechanical abrasion in combination with suction. Microdermabrasion treatments help to unclog congested pores and improve the appearance of dull skin. A series

Clear Tip #88:

Photodynamic Therapy can also be used to help clear back and body acne.

of microdermabrasion treatments can help to reduce the appearance of discoloration, mild acne scarring and mild fine lines. Microdermabrasion, combined with other treatments such as chemical peels, can improve the appearance of post-inflammatory hyperpigmentation (dark spots) after acne. Patients with very shallow scarring may notice improvement, but most patients with pitted acne scars will benefit more from laser resurfacing treatments than from microdermabrasion.

77. Which laser acne treatments are best for teenagers?

Photodynamic Therapy and the Isolaz® treatment are both very effective and safe laser acne treatments for teenagers. Photodynamic Therapy (or PDT) is not only anti-bacterial, but it is one of the only acne treatments that can decrease sebum production in teenage patients with oily skin. The Isolaz® treatment cleans out clogged pores and kills the P. acnes bacteria residing in the pores. In our experience, these laser treatments work best in combination with each other to produce long lasting results.

Clear Tip #89:

Try not to switch skin doctors too often if you can help it. Consistency to one provider will bring in better results in the long term most of the time.

78. Is photodynamic therapy safe in darker skinned patients?

When performed properly, photodynamic therapy is safe and effective for darker skinned patients. The aminolevulinic acid incubation time (the time the medicine stays on the skin) and the blue LED light treatment time may be shorter for patients with skin of color. Patients with skin of color must be very careful to avoid sun exposure after their photodynamic therapy treatment, so as to avoid post-inflammatory hyperpigmentation due to enhanced sun sensitivity from the aminolevulinic acid. However, when used correctly photodynamic therapy has actually been shown to treat PIH and help get rid of those pesky darks spots.[18]

79. What prescription medications are safe during pregnancy?

Prescription medications, labeled "category B" for pregnancy, are considered safe to use while you are pregnant. Pregnancy category B means that either 1) a medication has been studied in animals and no fetal effects were found but human first trimester studies are not available to confirm. 2) No evidence of risk in second

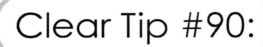

Clear Tip #90:

There are several acne imitators such as rosacea and pityrosporum folliculitis. If your acne is not responding to traditional therapy or is new in onset, be sure that your dermatologist considers another diagnosis.

and third trimester human studies or 3) fetal harm is possible but unlikely. Topical azelaic acid and topical clindamycin are both in this category and are used safely and successfully in our pregnant patient population for the treatment of acne. However, it is best to check with your obstetrician prior to using any medications while you are pregnant.

80. Why do acne scars develop?

Acne scars can develop after inflammatory acne. They are a result of a loss of collagen in an area that had acne as a result of a strong inflammatory reaction. Acne scars are more likely to develop on those who pick and pop their active acne lesions.

81. Why do some people get acne scars and other people don't?

Scar development can be influenced by many things, one of them being genetic. We find that some people are just prone to acne scarring and develop a pitted acne scar from even mild acne. We often see this running in families. For this reason, it is important to begin an acne-fighting regimen as soon as acne presents, in order to

Clear Tip #91:

PRP or Platelet Rich Plasma can be injected into acne scars immediately after fractional laser surgery to improve final result.

avoid future potentially scar-causing breakouts. Not all patients get scarring and sometimes it is hard to predict which patient will be left with residual scars from acne. This is why it's important for even mild acne to be treated promptly by a dermatologist. Starting an acne regimen early can eliminate the acne lesions before they lead to scarring. It is also helpful to avoid picking at acne and popping acne at home, as this type of manipulation may increase the likelihood of scarring.

82. What are the different types of acne scars?

The most common types of acne scars are atrophic, and hypertrophic scars. Atrophic scars are shallow pitted scars with smooth borders. Ice pick scars are a specific type of atrophic scar; ice pick scars are deep, pitted scars with very sharp borders. Hypertrophic scars are less common on the face than atrophic scars, we often see them on the back and chest. Hypertrophic scars are raised scars that are palpable above the skin's surface.

83. How can I remove the red marks left behind after adult acne?

Post-inflammatory erythema, or the red marks left

Clear Tip #92:

Topical dapsone (Aczone®) is a good topical acne medication to consider if you are sensitive to benzoyl peroxide.

behind after acne, can be treated with the KTP or V-Beam laser. Two or three treatments with the KTP laser are usually sufficient for greatly reducing the post-inflammatory erythema.

84. What causes "post-inflammatory hyperpigmentation"?

Post-inflammatory hyperpigmentation (PIH) results from an increase of skin pigment production after some injury or stress on the skin. Post-inflammatory hyperpigmentation often forms after an inflammatory reaction in the skin, like acne. In layman's terms, PIH is when the skin becomes discolored or darkened in an area that was recently inflamed-like a painful acne cyst. Inflammatory acne lesions can cause post-inflammatory hyperpigmentation, particularly in skin of color. We tell our patients that it is like the ashes after a fire. The fire was the breakout (inflammatory acne) and the ashes are remnants of the fire (PIH) that indicate where the pimples used to be. These ashes can sometime stick around for many months without treatment.

Clear Tip #93:

For patients who are prone to ingrown hairs, try shaving after showering. The steam will help soften the skin and make razor bumps less likely.

85. How long does PIH stay after acne has resolved?

Post-inflammatory hyperpigmentation (PIH) can improve with time, but without treatment it may linger for 6-12 months or longer. Topical prescription medications, such as hydroquinone, azeleic acid and tazarotene can be used to improve the appearance of PIH. Chemical peels and laser treatments, such as the Fractional Erbium Glass laser (Fraxel®), are very effective in treating PIH.

86. Will acne scars go away over time?

Atrophic acne scars, which have the appearance of a sunken recess, or a pit, in the skin, usually do not improve over time without treatment. However, lasers such as the fractional CO_2 laser and the Erbium Glass fractionated laser (Fraxel® laser) can stimulate the production of collagen to smooth out the pitted areas.

87. Are there any creams that treat acne scars?

In our experience, pitted acne scars do not improve much with use of topical creams only. Retinoids can stimulate collagen production, but rarely to a degree that is able to repair the pitted areas of acne scarring. Residual dark marks (called post-inflammatory hyperpigmentation)

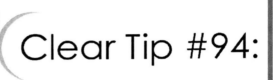

Clear Tip #94:

Subcision before acne scar laser surgery may help improve final results.

left behind after acne can sometimes be treated with creams such as hydroquinone, retinoids or azeleic acid. If the dark spots don't resolve after use of these creams, the Fraxel® laser or chemical peels can improve the remaining dark spots.

88. How soon after taking Accutane® can acne scars be treated?

Patients taking Accutane® experience impaired skin healing and light sensitivity, these qualities continue for months after Accutane® is discontinued. Depending on your skin type, dose of Accutane®, and the treatment modality chosen for treatment of acne scarring, your dermatologist will recommend an appropriate timeline for beginning treatment of acne scars. Standard guidelines are to wait six months after completion of Accutane® to initiate acne scar laser therapy.

89. What is the best laser treatment for acne scars?

In our opinion, the best lasers for the treatment of acne scars are the fractionated resurfacing lasers. The fractional CO_2 laser therapy is the most aggressive laser acne scar treatment available today. It produces

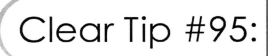

Clear Tip #95:

Patients with keratosis pilaris (bumps on upper arms) will often benefit by using a peel pad that contains salicylic and glycolic acid daily.

excellent results in one treatment, but patients must plan for four to five days of downtime after their treatment. The fractional erbium glass (Fraxel re:store®) laser produces similar results after a series of four treatments, though each treatment has only two to three days of downtime.

90. What is the Fractional CO2 laser?

The fractional CO_2 (carbon dioxide) laser is an effective laser for the treatment of acne scars. The newer "fractional" technology treats only a fraction of the skin, leaving healthy intact skin surrounding the treatment area. This allows for fast healing and very safe treatments for most skin types. The fractional CO_2 laser pokes small microscopic holes in the deeper layers of the skin. This process leads to the generation of new, healthy collagen to smooth out the acne scars. Improvement in acne scars can be seen in as early as one week following the fractional CO_2 laser treatment. Improvements in acne scarring will continue for up to six months following the initial treatment. Approximately 43-80% improvement of acne scarring is seen after 2 or 3 treatments, though results vary by the individual[19].

Clear Tip #96:

Don't use too many acne products at once. This can lead to irritation and confusion over which one is working.

91. What is the Fraxel® laser?

Fraxel® laser is the most well-known example of a fractional erbium glass laser; because the term Fraxel® is more well-known, we will refer to this laser as the Fraxel®. The Fraxel® is a non-ablative fractional laser treatment that is often used in the treatment of acne scarring. It is named the "Fraxel" since it only treats a small fraction of the skin each visit, leaving healthy skin between the treatment areas in order to decrease healing time. The Fraxel® laser uses microscopic columns of laser energy to penetrate into the skin's deeper layers in order to stimulate your body's own healing process. This stimulates the body to produce healthy collagen in order to repair the damaged skin. The Fraxel® treatment can smooth out acne scars in addition to treating the red and brown marks often left behind after acne lesions. The Fraxel® laser does not break the skin so it has less downtime than the fractional CO_2 laser, but usually requires four treatments instead of one.

92. What is the KTP laser?

The KTP laser is used to treat many causes of redness on the face, including blood vessels, rosacea and post-

Clear Tip #97:

Don't wash your skin too aggressively. Remember it is not dirt that causes acne and too much washing can lead to irritation.

inflammatory erythema (the redness left behind after acne). KTP is an abbreviation for potassium titanyl-phosphate, though the laser is commonly called the KTP laser. The KTP laser can significantly improve red acne scars after one to three treatments. It is not painful and there is no downtime after the treatments. Some improvement is seen very soon after the treatment and some improvement is seen in the weeks after the initial treatment. The KTP laser targets the hemoglobin (red) areas on the skin. The energy of the KTP laser causes the blood vessels just below the skin's surface to collapse. The collapsing of the blood vessels decreases the red appearance of the acne scars left behind after the acne clears.

93. Can the Vbeam® laser be used to treat red marks from recent acne?

Yes, the Vbeam® laser can be used to treat red marks from recent acne. The Vbeam® works similarly to the KTP laser, and they are both vascular lasers. This means that the Vbeam® targets the hemoglobin (red cells) in the skin, which causes the tiny blood vessels that contribute to the appearance of redness to collapse.

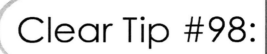

Clear Tip #98:

Always bring a list of your past medications (both prescription and non-prescription) to your first dermatologist appointment.

94. Is laser treatment of acne scars permanent?

Laser treatment of acne scars stimulates new collagen production in the skin, to smooth out the skin's surface. The results are permanent.

95. How long after fractional CO_2 laser treatment do acne scars improve?

Some improvement of acne scars is seen as early as one week after fractional CO_2 laser treatment. Collagen production continues for up to six months after the initial treatment, so the acne scars continue to improve as time goes on.

96. How much downtime is there after fractional CO_2 laser treatment?

Depending on the laser, fractional CO_2 lasers usually have about 3-6 days of downtime after the procedure. During this time, the skin is healing from the wound the laser caused in order to stimulate collagen remodeling. During the healing period, we often recommend patients apply Aquaphor ointment to speed up recovery time.

Clear Tip #99:

When using a topical retinoind, start out 2 or 3 times per week applying just a pea sized amount to your forehead, cheeks and chin. Then increase to more often if tolerated well.

97. Does my acne need to be completely clear prior to having laser treatment for acne scars?

Acne scars may be treated once the acne is mostly improved, though acne does not need to be completely clear prior to treatment. For some patients, if they were to wait until their acne was 100% clear, they would never be able to address acne scars.

98. Can fillers be used to treat acne scars?

Dermal fillers can be used to treat acne scars temporarily. Fillers, such as Restylane®, Juvederm® and Perlane®, can be injected directly into the pitted area. They help to add volume where volume has been lost from scarring, and can often even out pitted rolling scars. However, dermal fillers do not actually change the scars, they merely camouflage them. Dermal fillers are a great quick fix, but the results last only six to twelve months. For patients who don't mind the upkeep, dermal fillers may be a good option for the treatment of acne scars.

99. What is the CROSS technique of treating acne scars?

The CROSS technique uses very high concentrations

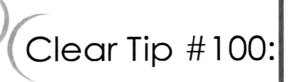

Clear Tip #100:

Knowledge is power: The more you know about acne and its treatments, the better chance of success you will have.

of TCA acid, which is applied directly into the atrophic (or "pitted") scar. This process is meant to stimulate collagen remodeling in the area and smooth out the acne scar. We prefer using laser therapy to treat acne scars because we find the results to be more consistent.

100. What is the F.A.S.T.® procedure for acne scars?

The F.A.S.T.® procedure for acne scars targets localized areas of acne scarring, rather than treating the entire face. F.A.S.T.® is an acronym for Focal Acne Scar Treatment. Traditional methods of fractional CO_2 laser resurfacing for acne scars utilized "medium" strength energy over the entire face. Dr. Schweiger developed F.A.S.T.® as a method of treating acne scars with higher energy levels, but having a shorter healing time. The F.A.S.T.® procedure uses the "fraction of a fraction" idea; not only is the laser fractionated, but only a fraction of the skin is being treated at a time. Results have been excellent, with most patients seeing between 50-70% improvement of their acne scars with just 3-4 days of downtime.

PART 6
TOP 100
ACNE-FIGHTING TIPS

This section conveniently lists all of the acne tips placed throughout the book, making them easily accessable for future reference.

1. Don't pop pimples at home – this can cause more inflammation on the skin.

2. Visit your dermatologist as soon as acne develops; delaying treatment for even mild acne can lead to scarring.

3. Laser and light treatments are great for teenagers who forget to apply medications.

4.   Wear loose cotton clothing while working out, to help prevent body acne.

5.   Wash your clothes on a regular basis. Wearing the same outfit for extended periods of time may promote bacteria growth.

6.   Washing with a salicylic acid cleanser after working out can help to prevent body acne.

7.   Make sure to change your pillowcase every day when acne is a consideration. Dead skin cells, dirt and debris accumulate on the pillowcases and can lead to more breakouts.

8.   If you're running out of clean pillowcases, then use a clean t-shirt as a pillowcase alternative.

9.   Use a white pillowcase if you use benzoyl peroxide at night; it can bleach fabric, but won't bleach your skin.

10.   Avoid hairstyles that require a lot of hair product, as oils can clog pores.

11.   If you're using hairspray or other product on your hair, sleep with a headband on to keep it off your face.

12.   A low glycemic diet may help to reduce acne. Cut back on processed foods and add more leafy green vegetables and berries to your diet.

Low Glycemic Foods:	High Glycemic Foods:
Carrots	Alcohol
Broccoli	Pineapple
Cauliflower	Pasta
Lettuce	Pizza
Red Peppers	Bagels
Eggplant	White Bread
Mushrooms	Potato Chips
Whole Wheat	Corn Chips
Oat Bran	Cake
All-Bran	Pancakes
Sweet Potatoes	Waffles
Whole Milk	Soda
Soy Milk	Candy Bars
Chick Peas	Sweetened beverages
Kidney Beans	French Fries
Haricot Vert	White Rice
Lentils	Tapioca
Yellow Split Peas	Pretzels
Hummus	Scones
Walnuts	Muffins
Cashews	Rice Cakes
Peanuts	Sugared Cereals

13. Choose organic milk when possible, there is less of a chance that the cow has been injected with hormones, which could potentially lead to acne breakouts.

14. Adults with acne can benefit from a retinoid—it helps treat acne and wrinkles.

15. Wear sunscreen daily while taking oral antibiotics for acne.

16. For sun protection, we recommend using a physical sunblock containing zinc oxide or titanium dioxide; chemical sunscreens are more likely to irritate.

17. If you have a pimple and need it gone fast, see your dermatologist for a cortisone injection, which can flatten your pimple in 24 hours, and is usually covered by insurance.

18. Stress can be a contributor to acne outbreaks. Try to exercise on a daily basis. A workout, when combined with meditation or some other form of relaxation, can help decrease stress.

19. If it doesn't seem like acne, it might actually be something else such as rosacea or Pityrosporum follicultitis. Talk to your dermatologist about other diagnoses that look similar to acne.

20.   Blue and red light therapy are safe and effective acne treatment options during pregnancy.

21. Glycolic and lactic acid cleansers can safely be used during pregnancy.

22.   Acne-like bumps on the beard are not always acne – it may be a condition called pseudofolliculitis barbae. Consult your dermatologist if you're not sure.

23.   Less is more: even over-the-counter formulations can cause excessive dryness if overused. Take a few days off from your acne products if you develop redness or irritation.

24.   Look at your skin care products and if they contain fragrance it may be time to look for a different brand. Synthetic fragrances contain many ingredients that may be irritating to your skin.

25.   Make sure all of your skincare products say "non-comedogenic" or "non-acnegenic" on the label somewhere.

26.   Use a pea-size amount of your acne medication, to minimize risk of skin irritation and apply to the whole face: cheeks, forehead and temple. Don't just spot treat!

27.   Apply moisturizer before and after using a topical retinoid. This technique is called "sandwiching"

and helps cut down on irritation to the skin.

28. Apply retinoids in the evening to reduce sun sensitivity.

29. While taking Accutane®, apply Aquaphor® ointment liberally to your lips, to avoid excessive dryness.

30. Use an at-home blue light device between in-office blue light treatments for best results.

31. Avoid sun exposure for 48 hours after photodynamic therapy.

32. Use a foaming cleanser that doesn't need to be rubbed into the skin to lather. Rubbing the skin can cause further irritation.

33. Don't do bathroom surgery! Rather than perform extractions at home, book an appointment with a medically trained skincare professional who uses sterile tools to minimize risk and maximize results.

34. Stay away from spa facials where the esthetician is massaging oils and heavy creams into your face.

35. If you have a tendency to pick and squeeze your pimples, avoid looking into mirrors during the day.

36. Wash your washcloths often so you're not touching your skin with bacteria trapped in the towel.

37. Make sure to wash your hands before applying

your makeup. The oils and bacteria on your fingers may be contributing to your acne breakouts.

38. Don't sleep in your makeup. If you're too tired to wash your face, use a makeup remover pad.

39. Wipe your cell phone down daily with an alcohol swab to kill any bacteria and reduce oils that may get transferred onto your skin.

40. Swap your cream blush for a powder blush. Cream formulations are more likely to consist of pore-clogging ingredients.

41. Make sure to wash your makeup brushes on a regular basis to clear them of bacteria and debris that can lead to acne breakouts.

42. Stop using retinoids three days prior to laser scar resurfacing treatments.

43. Visualize a stop sign to help yourself put the brakes on negative thoughts about yourself.

44. Don't use your fingertips to wash your face, as bacteria lurking under the nail can aggravate acne.

45. To avoid skin picking, time yourself in the bathroom so you're not allowing yourself extra time to pick.

46. Avoid touching your face when working or

studying for exams. Face touching leads to breakouts.

47.   Wash your hands before washing your face.

48.   Strongly consider Photodynamic Therapy or Accutane® if you have severe acne.

49.   Remember that even celebrities get acne. Cameron Diaz, Annalynne McCord, Kate Hudson have all had bouts with acne.

50.   Don't fight acne alone—partner with a skincare professional, such as a dermatologist.

51.   Don't waste your time on microdermabrasion if you have deep pitted scars

52. If your skin is feeling dry, skip your acne medications for a day then restart. (Don't forget to moisturize though).

53. Rosacea patients can often benefit from sulfur based washes.

54. Always give your new acne regimen at least 2 months to work before you change it.

55. Keep a diary of past medications so you will be able to look up what worked and what didn't in case you forget (as everyone does).

56. Use mineral based make-up to cover up an outbreak.

57. Men can use tinted moisturizer to cover up a break out.

58. Don't stop using acne medications just because you are clear.

59. Hormonal acne in females can often be treated successfully with birth control or Spironolactone (both are prescription, so see your doctor!)

60. Laser Genesis is a good treatment for mild acne scars.

61. Not all fractionated laser used in acne scars are the same. Make sure to ask your dermatologist the difference before you get treatment.

62. Do not wait to "outgrow" acne, seek treatment now.

63. One size does not fit all for acne treatment. Make sure you have a customized regimen.

64. Keeping pictures of your face can be a great way to track your progress.

65. Check out ClearTrack™ at www.clearclinic.com to easily track your progress on your way to clear skin.

66. Avoid alcohol if you are taking oral antibiotics or Accutane®.

67. If you are overweight, try to get back to your ideal

weight. Obesity is associated with increased acne.

68. Seeking aggressive treatment for acne early can decrease the chance of having scars later.

69. Consider a Fraxel® treatment if you have post-inflammatory hyper-pigmentation (residual dark spots after acne resolves).

70. Both green tea and tea tree oil are good natural ingredients that may help fight acne.

71. Consider KTP laser treatment if you have red marks from old acne.

72. If you decide to do laser resurfacing for acne scars, give yourself about 7 days to be out of sight if you can.

73. Your acne does not need to be completely clear before treating scars.

74. Chemical peels are not usually the best treatment for deep acne scars.

75. If you use benzoyl peroxide, make sure it is micronized. It can then be absorbed better.

76. If you have dry skin, use a moisturizer cream; if you have oily skin use a moisturizer lotion instead.

77. Consider a live video chat with a Personal Acne Coach™ if you do not have easy access to a

dermatologist: www.clearclinic.com.

78. Don't share acne medications with your friends.

79. F.A.S.T.® Laser Treatments are a great way to reduce acne scars. Patients can fly into NYC for treatment and have their travel costs included: www.flyinforclearskin.com.

80. If you are on Benzamycin®, keep it in the fridge or it will stop working as well after a few weeks.

81. Do not use expired acne medication, if it is old throw it out!

82. If you pick your skin and it starts bleeding put Aquaphor® ointment on the wound to prevent a scab from forming. (And try not to do that again!)

83. Make sure you have a spot treatment in your regimen.

84. We often recommend patients with chronic psuedofolliculitis barbae (razor bumps), consider laser hair removal as a permanent treatment option.

85. A monthly mask can sometimes boost your acne-fighting regimen!

86. Do not pick at your skin if it is flaky from too much medication use. Instead use extra moisturizer that day.

87. Acne can occur on the buttock and legs, and

those areas often do well with a benzoyl peroxide wash.

88. Photodynamic Therapy can also be used to help clear back and body acne.

89. Try not to switch skin doctors too often if you can help it. Consistency to one provider will bring in better results in the long term most of the time.

90. There are several acne imitators such as rosacea and pityrosporum folliculitis. If your acne is not responding to traditional therapy or is new in onset, be sure that your dermatologist considers another diagnosis.

91. PRP or Platelet Rich Plasma can be injected into acne scars immediately after fractional laser surgery to improve final result.

92. Topical dapsone (Aczone®) is a good topical acne medication to consider if you are sensitive to benzoyl peroxide.

93. For patients who are prone to ingrown hairs, try shaving after showering. The steam will help soften the skin and make razor bumps less likely.

94. Subscision before acne scar laser surgery helps improve final results in our opinion.

95. Patients with keratosis pilaris (bumps on upper

arms) will often benefit by using a peel pad that contains salicylic and glycolic acid daily.

96. Don't use too many acne products at once. This can lead to irritation and confusion over which one is working.

97. Don't wash your skin too aggressively. Remember it is not dirt that causes acne and too much washing can lead to irritation.

98. Always bring a list of your past medications (both prescription and non-prescription) to your first dermatologist appointment.

99. When using a topical retinoind, start out 2 or 3 times per week applying just a pea sized amount to your forehead, cheeks and chin. Then increase to more often if tolerated well.

100. Knowledge is power: The more you know about acne and its treatments, the better chance of success you will have.

Your Future is Clear

Congratulations, you just completed the first step towards clear skin. As you now know, acne can and does affect every single one of us at some point in our lives. Whether you're a teenager or an adult, light or dark skinned, acne breakouts can occur at any time and often pop up seemingly out of nowhere. We hope this book has helped eliminate the mystery from acne breakouts. Instead of just accepting your fate, we hope you've become empowered after reading this book and will fight acne head on; knowing that achieving clear skin is not only a possibility but it is attainable.

Studies have shown that over 80% of acne sufferers do not see a dermatologist for treatment. However, we recommend all acne patients partner with a board-certified dermatologist whenever possible to optimize care. We encourage you to visit the American Academy of Dermatology website at www.aad.org to find a dermatologist in your area, or if you are in New York we would be happy to treat you ourselves in one of our offices. If you do not have access to a dermatologist, Clear Clinic is proud to offer a new service where certified skincare professionals (Personal Acne Coaches®) can assess you online and help determine if you need to be under the care of a dermatologist, or if over-the-counter treatments may work for you. For patients who are candidates for over-the-counter treatment, a personalized treatment regimen is then put together. To read more about this program please visit www.clearclinic.com.

With the knowledge you have uncovered in this book, you will now be an active participant in your treatment plan, which ultimately sets you up for success. We'd love to hear from you on your road to clear, acne-free skin. Drop us a line and tell us all about your progress at mystory@clearclinic.com.

Glossary

Acne: Acne (also known as acne vulgaris) is a common skin condition made up of one or more lesions scattered on the face, back, chest, buttocks, or anywhere on the body where sebaceous glands and hair follicles exist. Acne can appear in many different forms including: open comedones (blackheads), closed comedones (whiteheads), papules (red bumps), pustules (pus bumps), and cysts (painful deep nodules).

Acne Scars: Residual damage to the skin results from inflammatory acne vulgaris. Often described as "ice pick" or "rolling," these scars are permanent and can only be changed by physical treatments. When the body has a vigorous response, almost inappropriately strong, to acne bacteria, this can lead to inflammation. Intense inflammation over time can cause scarring. Some people are more prone to scarring than others. Some patients with intense inflammation can end up with significant scars.

Astringent: Also known as toner, used to remove excess oil and dirt from the skin.

Atrophic Scars: A type of acne scar more common on the face. Atrophic means there has been a loss of tissue and a pitted mark is left behind.

Benzoyl Peroxide: A common ingredient in many acne-fighting products that works as an antimicrobial to help kill P. acnes bacteria and improve acne lesions such as papules and pustules.

Blackhead: Open comedone with no inflammation. Can be raised or flat on the skin and center is darker. Contains clogged pore filled with sebum, dead cells and sometimes bacteria. The surface is black because the contents inside became oxidized from the outside air.

Blue Light Therapy: Blue light is a physical acne treatment that works by directly killing the acne causing bacteria, Propionibacterium Acnes (P. Acnes). Blue light is often administered through LED lights. It can be performed in office and at home through handheld devices.

Chemical Peels: A treatment performed in a dermatologist's office that is aimed to treat fine lines, pigment (brown spots), photo-damage, melasma, active acne and sometimes acne scars. The process involves applying a chemical agent to the skin for a specified amount of time in order to remove the epidermis (top layer of skin) and stimulate collagen remodeling.

Fractional CO2: A safe and effective treatment for the

majority of patients with acne scars. This laser pokes tiny microscopic holes in the skin down past the epidermis and into the dermis. These holes cause new collagen to be generated, which fills in the acne scars and creates rejuvenated smoother skin.

Clarisonic®: Home mechanical brush device used daily to remove oil, debris, and makeup. Can prevent acne breakouts and remove dead cells and sebum, which can cause pimples.

Cortisone Injection: A brief in-office treatment performed to quickly reduce the appearance of active acne. A medication called triamcinolone is injected at a low concentration directly into an inflammatory papule or cyst (aka "pimple"). This procedure takes only a minute and is relatively pain-free. Over the next 24 hours, the pimple will improve significantly and flatten out. This is the most effective spot treatment for active acne.

Cyst: A nodule below the skin in the dermis, which is filled with blood, bacteria and/or pus. May become painful and inflamed (red) which may require extraction, drainage, excision or a cortisone injection.

Dead Skin Cells: Layers of the epidermis that are constantly renewing. The top, superficial layer sheds and the bottom layers of the epidermis rise to the stop to continue the cycle. Dead skin cells sometimes stick inside the pores, forming plugs that can lead to acne.

Dermis: The deeper layer of skin, located under the epidermis (the top layer of skin). Where hair follicles, sebaceous glands and fibroblasts are located. Gives strength and elasticity to the skin.

Epidermis: Top layer of skin, supported by the underlying dermis. The outermost layer of the epidermis is made up of dead skin cells, which rise to the top and flake off.

Exfoliation: The process of removing dead skin cells chemically (such as chemical peels or peel pads) or physically (such as microscrubs or microdermabrasion).

Extractions: A method that manually removes sebum, dead cells and bacteria from within blocked pores. Often performed by a licensed esthetician or medical provider. Often includes steaming prior to open pores and cotton tip applicators, comedone extractor or small needle remove blackheads and whiteheads.

F.A.S.T.®: Developed by Dr. Eric Schweiger, F.A.S.T.® is an acronym for Focal Acne Scar Treatment. This procedure utilizes very high laser energy levels of the fractional CO_2 laser to focally treat only the scarred areas, while leaving the normal surrounding skin intact. The new technique allows for improved efficacy, faster healing time and increased patient satisfaction. All F.A.S.T.® procedures include a Fraxel® laser treatment approximately 6 weeks after Fractional CO_2 treatment, to further reduce the scarring and improve skin texture.

Fraxel®: Brand name of an Erbium Fractionated Laser. This non-invasive laser treatment can be used to treat fine lines, wrinkles, sun damage, blood vessels, acne scars, and melasma. It was named "Fraxel" because it only treats a fraction of the skin, leaving normal skin in between treated areas to speed up healing time.

Hair Follicle: Small channel where hair grows. Opens up to the surface of a pore. Can be blocked by multiple hairs, bacteria or pus.

Hypertrophic Scars: A type of acne scar more common on the back and chest. These scars are thick and lumpy and sit above the surface of the skin.

Ice Pick Scar: Scar resulting from inflammatory acne. Narrow craters in the skin that appear like a needle or puncture. Often needs laser resurfacing to stimulate collagen to help decrease appearance.

Isolaz®: An acne treatment designed to clean out your pores and destroy the bacteria that causes acne. In this treatment, a gentle vacuum cleans your pores, while pulsed light simultaneously kills the acne bacteria and decreases inflammation. Safe for all skin types, it treats inflammatory acne, as well as comedones and milder acne. Isolaz® can also be used for the maintenance therapy.

KTP Laser: KTP stands for Potassium Titanyl-

Phosphate. The KTP laser is used to treat blood vessels on the face, redness from rosacea and post inflammatory erythema.

Laser Genesis®: A laser treatment best used in a series that can improve the appearance of the skin. Laser Genesis uses a short-pulsed 1064nm non-ablative laser to minimize pores, reduce acne, improve superficial acne scars, and decrease generalized redness.

Levulan®: The brand of a topical medication known as 5-aminolevulinic acid. This photosensitizing agent is applied to the skin in photodynamic therapy. This acid is pain free on application and causes the skin to become receptive to an activating light source.

Microdermabrasion: An office-based procedure that uses gentle mechanical abrasion combined with suction to remove the outermost layer of dead skin. Often used in acne patients to remove blackheads and whiteheads.

Papule: A round elevation of skin less than 1cm, often with no visible fluid or pus. Can be brown, purple, pink or red in color. Often tender.

Photodynamic Therapy (PDT): A non-invasive therapy that utilizes blue light treatment in combination with the application of the photosensitizing agent, typically aminolevulinic acid (brand name Levulan®). PDT has also been shown to be a safe and effective treatment for acne by shrinking oil glands and killing the acne bacteria.

Post Inflammatory Hyperpigmentation: Darkening of the skin occurring after inflammation or damage to the skin, such as an acne cyst or trauma or manipulation to the skin. Can last weeks to months and fades slowly, and can be treated by peels, creams or laser therapy. This condition is more common in darker skin patients.

Post-Inflammatory Erythema: Redness occurring on the skin at the site of trauma or manipulation. Often occurs after an acne cyst or pimple. Can occur after manual manipulation of the skin. Generally fades over time, but can be decreased by laser therapy. This condition is more common in lighter skin patients.

Pustule: A small, round elevated bump on the skin, which contains pus. Can be opened or extracted by a dermatologist or medical provider.

Red Light Therapy: A light treatment used for reducing inflammation. Red light can help speed up healing time post procedures and can decease post-inflammatory erythema associated with acne.

Rolling Scars: Depressed, atrophic acne scars on the skin that have a wavy texture.

Sebaceous Gland: Small gland in the skin that secretes a yellow oil matter called sebum, which hydrates and makes the skin waterproof. Often collects bacteria and can be the initial site of cyst formation.

Smoothbeam®: An in office laser treatment that targets and heats collagen in the dermis. This procedure applies thermal energy directly to the sebaceous glands and destroys the bacteria that cause acne. The thermal injury changes the structure of the sebaceous glans and helps with long-term reduction of acne.

Tanda® Blue Light: At home blue light therapy designed to kill the P. acne bacteria that cause acne breakouts. Can be used for maintenance in any acne regimen.

Tria® Blue Light Handheld Device: At home blue light therapy designed to penetrate deep within the skin to eliminate acne-causing bacteria and help prevent future breakouts. Often used as maintenance therapy for patients doing in office physical therapies but can also be used on its own.

Whitehead: Closed comedone containing bacteria, sebum, oil and dead cells. No inflammation is present. Pore remains white as it is covered by a layer of skin and not exposed to air.

1. Yosipovitch G et al, "Study of psychological stress, sebum production and acne vulgaris in adolescents," *Acta Dermato-Venereologica,* 2007.

2. Rouhani P, et al "Acne improves with a popular, low glycemic diet from South Beach," *Journal of the American Academy of Dermatology* 2009; 60(suppl): Abstract P706.

3. Goldberg J, Dabade T et al, "Changing Age of Acne Vulgaris Visits: Another Sign of Earlier Puberty?" *Pediatric Dermatology*, November/ December 2011.

4. Collier CN et al, "The prevalence of acne in adults 20 years and older," *Journal of the American Academy of Dermatology*, Oct 2007.

5. Perkins AC et al, "Acne Vulgaris in Women: Prevalence Across the Life Span," *Journal of Women's Health*, Feb 2012.

6. Saitta P, Keehan P et al, "An update on the presence of psychiatric comorbitidies in acne patients, part 1: overview of prevalence," *Cutis*, July 2011.

7. Saitta P, Keehan P, et al, "An update on the presence of psychiatric comorbidities in acne patients, part 2: depression, anxiety, and suicide," *Cutis*, Aug 2011.

8. Narahari S et al, "What's new in antibiotics in the management of acne?" *G Ital Dermatol Venereol*, June 2012.

9. Hull PR, Demkiw-Bartel C, "Isotretinoin use in acne: prospective evaluation of adverse events," *Journal of Cutaneous Medicine and Surgery*, April 2000.

10. Rademaker M, "Adverse effects of isotretinoin: A retrospective review of 1743 patients started

on isotretinoin," *Australasian Journal of Dermatology*, November 2010.

11. Halvorsen JA et al, "Suicidal ideation, mental health problems, and social impairment are increased in adolescents with acne: a population-based study," *Journal of Investigative Dermatology*, February 2011.

12. Misery L, "Consequences of psychological distress in adolescents with acne," *Journal of Investigative Dermatology*, February 2011.

13. Crockett SD et al, "Isotretinoin use and the risk of inflammatory bowel disease: a case-control study," *The American Journal of Gastroenterology*, September 2010.

14. Block SG et al, "Exacerbation of facial acne vulgaris after consuming pure chocolate," *Journal of the American Academy of Dermatology*, Oct 2011.

15. Halvorson JA et al, "A Population-Based Study of Acne and Body Mass Index in Adolescents," *Archives of Dermatology*, Jan 2012.

16. Rouhani P et al, "Acne improves with a popular, low glycemic diet from South Beach," *Journal of the American Academy of Dermatology*, Mar 2009.

17. Adebamowo CA et al, "High school dietary intake and teenage acne," *Journal of the American Academy of Dermatology*, Feb 2005.

18. Kumaresan M and Srinivas CR, "Efficacy of IPL in the treatment of acne vulgaris: comparison of single- and burst-pulse mode in IPL," *Indian Journal of Dermatology*, Oct-Dec 2010.

19. Gold MH and Biron J, "Efficacy of a novel combination of pneumatic energy and broadband light for the treatment of acne," *Journal of Drugs*

and Dermatology, July 2008.

20. Terrell S, Aires D, Schweiger ES. "Treatment of acne vulgaris using blue light photodynamic therapy in an African-American patient." *J Drugs Dermatol*. July 2009.

21. Chapas AM, Brightman L et al, "Successful treatment of acneiform scarring with CO2 ablative fractional resurfacing," *Lasers in Surgery and Medicine*, Aug 2008.

CPSIA information can be obtained at www.ICGtesting.com
Printed in the USA
LVOW11s1453140515

438528LV00016B/322/P

9 780615 889689